Health Benefits of Vitamin K_2

A Revolutionary Natural Treatment for Heart Disease and Bone Loss

Larry M. Howard
& Anthony G. Payne, Ph.D.

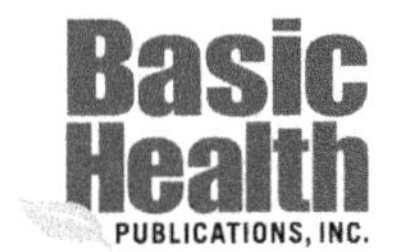

The information contained in this book is based upon the research and personal and professional experiences of the authors. It is not intended as a substitute for consulting with your physician or other healthcare provider. Any attempt to diagnose and treat an illness should be done under the direction of a healthcare professional.

The publisher does not advocate the use of any particular healthcare protocol but believes the information in this book should be available to the public. The publisher and authors are not responsible for any adverse effects or consequences resulting from the use of the suggestions, preparations, or procedures discussed in this book. Should the reader have any questions concerning the appropriateness of any procedures or preparation mentioned, the authors and the publisher strongly suggest consulting a professional healthcare advisor.

Basic Health Publications, Inc.
www.basichealthpub.com

Library of Congress Cataloging-in-Publication Data

Howard, Larry M.
Health benefits of vitamin K2 : a revolutionary natural treatment for heart disease and bone loss / Larry M. Howard and Anthony G. Payne.

p. cm.
ncludes bibliographical references and index.
ISBN: 978-1-59120-184-7 (Pbk.)
ISBN: 978-1-68162-731-1 (Hardcover)

1. Vitamin K2—Therapeutic use. 2. Heart—Diseases—Treatment.
3. Bone—Diseases—Treatment. I. Payne, Anthony G. II. Title.

QP772.V56H69 2006
612.3'99—dc22

2006018034

Editor: John Anderson ■ Copyeditor: Nancy Ringer
Typesetting and Book design: Gary A. Rosenberg
Cover Design: Mike Stromberg

Contents

Introduction

We have all read or heard stories about how we are on the cusp of one revolution or another in medicine and health care, or about the advent of some "miraculous" drug, product, or device. Some, if not most, of these turn out to be largely hype, while others are genuinely promising—and, yes, on occasion we see the debut of something that truly turns the tables on a human affliction or malady.

This holds true with respect to both pharmaceuticals and natural health products. For example, coenzyme Q_{10} (coQ_{10}) was discovered in the United States in 1957 by Professor Frederick Crane at the University of Wisconsin, and a year later its chemical structure was published. During the ensuing fifty years, a great many studies have been done, some in the United States and most in Japan, which have provided clear scientific evidence that coQ_{10} is of benefit in treating some forms of heart disease and cancer, as well as periodontal disease and more. A similar path from "lab novelty" to "scientifically validated" has attended s-adenosylmethionine (SAMe), a compound that relieves depression on par with Prozac.

Now we have menaquinone-7 (MK-7), a form of vitamin K_2 that laboratory studies and clinical trials indicate may be one of biomedicine's most powerful tools for halting and reversing bone loss, as well as for pulling calcium out of hardened arteries. No, it isn't a miracle by a long shot, but it appears to qualify as "near miraculous" in the sense that it is likely to put a significant dent in some major medical challenges of our time, such as osteoporosis and atherosclerosis.

In this book, you will learn what vitamin K_2 is and what it does, as well as how diet and lifestyle can complement its activity in your body. And in so doing, you will come to know how this compound can help you in your personal pursuit of one of humankind's most cherished and universal goals: to live a long high-quality life.

> *"The value of an idea lies in the using of it."*
> —Thomas Alva Edison (1847–1931)

1

What Is Vitamin K?

Vitamin K is critical for building and maintaining vibrant health. This vitamin performs two primary functions in our bodies: it is essential for healthy blood clotting and plays a vital role in maintaining strong and healthy bones. When it is deficient or not well utilized in our bodies, serious, life-threatening conditions and even death can result.

Unfortunately, our bodies store only limited amounts of vitamin K. Healthy bacteria living in our intestines produce much of the vitamin K we need. The rest of the vitamin K we require for optimal health must come from the foods we eat. Vitamin K deficiencies often go undetected and can escalate unnoticed, culminating in serious health conditions (see page 7); thus, it is paramount to keep a watchful eye out for deficiency symptoms in concert with receiving proper medical testing. Vitamin K deficiencies can be brought about by a number of factors, including poor diet, the use of certain prescription or illicit drugs, the long-term use of antibiotics, or certain genetic conditions and predispositions.

Recently, scientists have isolated specific compounds in vitamin K that appear to be the active players in generating its health benefits. One of the most effective components in the vitamin K family of compounds is menaquinone-7, also known as MK-7. The menaquinones in vitamin K have been studied extensively worldwide and offer the promise of preventing and even reversing specific diseases. MK-7, for example, has been shown in several

> MK-7 has been shown in several studies to reverse and even prevent some forms of cardiovascular disease by eliminating excess calcium in the blood. MK-7 is also effective in reversing osteoporosis.

studies to reverse and even prevent some forms of cardiovascular disease by eliminating excess calcium in the blood. In other studies, MK-4 and especially MK-7 have been shown to be effective in reversing osteoporosis. Furthermore, studies indicate that MK-7 may help lower cholesterol, play a role in preventing Alzheimer's disease, and treat some forms of cancer. Vitamin K is also a well-known and powerful antioxidant.

THE DISCOVERY OF VITAMIN K

In 1929, Danish scientist Henrik Dam discovered that when chicks were fed a fat-free diet, their blood began leaking out from various blood vessels. In addition, he observed that their blood-clotting abilities were seriously impaired. Closer scrutiny disclosed that the restricted diet also caused the reduction of a unique compound typically found in fat. Dam figured out that this compound was integral to the blood's ability to coagulate or clot normally. Dam dubbed this compound that promoted blood clotting the "koagulation vitamin," which later became known as vitamin K (for "koagulation"). Years of follow-up research verified its integral role in coagulation, among other vital functions in the body.

Although there are technically five forms of vitamin K, the name generally refers to three basic substances: K_1, known as phylloquinone; K_2, a group of compounds called the menaquinones; and a synthetic version known as K_3 or menadione. The natural K compounds are found in the fatty part of foods. For example, green vegetables (such as broccoli) and soybean, canola, sunflower, and other plant oils are good sources of vitamin K_1. Butter, some cheeses, chicken, liver, egg yolks, and fermented soybean foods contain K_2.

The K Family of Vitamins

Five different compounds, numbered one through five, make up the vitamin K family:

- **Vitamin K_1:** Phylloquinone (also known as methylphytyl naphthoquinone, phytonadione, phytomenadione, phytonadione, 2-methyl-3-phytyl-1-1, 4-naphthoquinone)—Used to treat and prevent hypoprothrombinemia (deficiency of prothrombin) and hemorrhagic disease. It is also prescribed as a supplement for people who take broad-spectrum antibiotics or oral anticoagulants in high doses or for prolonged periods of time. It can be used topically to treat burns and stretch marks.
- **Vitamin K_2:** Menaquinone 1 through 13 (also known as menatertenone)—Used in the prevention and treatment of bone loss and the reduction of calcification of the arteries. It may be supportive in reducing total cholesterol levels.
- **Vitamin K_3:** Menadione (also known as menadione sodium bisulfite, 2-methyl-1-4, 4-naphthoquinone)—Used primarily by the pet-food industry in animal feed.
- **Vitamin K_4:** Menadiol acetate (also known as menadiol diacetate, menadiol sodium diphosphate, menadiol sodium phosphate, menadiolum solubile methylnaphthohydroquinone)—Used to treat hypoprothrombinemia (deficiency of prothrombin) via injections.
- **Vitamin K_5:** 4-amino-2-methyl-1-naphthol—Used to inhibit the growth of fungi.

Unfortunately, the human body can store only a small amount of vitamin K, primarily in the liver. Consequently, consuming foods rich in vitamin K and ensuring that our bodies are producing adequate amounts of this compound will help support optimal health.

THE HEALTH BENEFITS OF VITAMIN K

Given its importance in health and healing, it follows that we need to maintain optimal levels of vitamin K in our bodies. Naturally, eating a balanced diet containing vitamin K–rich foods and taking a dietary supplement containing K is important. Nevertheless, the primary source for all forms of vitamin K is the friendly bacteria in our colons and intestinal tract.

This colony of "good" bacteria is vital to health and plays an important role in the proper function of our immune system. Good bacteria keep harmful bacteria and fungi under control in our bodies. "Bad" bacteria and fungi, like all living things, want to live and proliferate when they enter our bodies, but do so at our expense. Many people have a constant tug-of-war going on in their colons and intestines between the good bacteria and the disease-causing bacteria and fungi. As long as the good microorganisms win (and continue to make vitamin K in the process), we are more apt to remain healthy.

When we fail to get enough nutrients because of a poor diet, or when we use certain prescription drugs that deplete and inhibit our body's synthesis, absorption, or utilization of nutrients, the good bacteria begin to lose, thus bringing about conditions that can compromise the efficient operation of the immune system. When we take heavy doses of antibiotics, especially for extended periods of time, they destroy not only the bad bacteria but also the good bacteria that support the health of the body and produce vitamin K. For this reason, it is essential for people taking antibiotics to take measures to increase the healthy bacteria in the gut. Some of these measures include eating soy yogurt with live culture and drinking beverages rich in gut-friendly acidophilus. Taking probiotic nutritional supplements can also help.

Vitamin K absorption begins in the intestinal tract and colon, with intestinal absorption varying with solubility. Vitamin K_1 and K_2, for example, are adequately absorbed through the gastrointestinal tract providing that bile salts are present. These vitamins are then transported throughout the body, for the most part by way of the lymphatic system (which circulates lymph fluid throughout our bodies). Vitamin K_1 is absorbed primarily in the small intestine, whereas vitamin K_2 is absorbed in the small intestine and colon.

So, there is a dynamic interaction and interdependence between diet, dietary and supplement intake of vitamins K_1 and K_2, the integrity of the gut, the use of certain medications, and vitamin K status.

WHAT HAPPENS WHEN WE DON'T GET ENOUGH VITAMIN K?

Vitamin K deficiency is a very serious matter and should not be taken lightly. The diet of people in most Western societies provides adequate levels of vitamin K. However, when practices that erode the absorption and availability of vitamin K—such as prescription or illegal drug use or excessive use of over-the-counter aspirin or, especially, anticoagulants—are factored in, vitamin K status can be compromised. When this occurs, it becomes important to supplement with the right kind and amounts of vitamin K.

The following ailments have been linked to vitamin K deficiencies:

- Anemia
- Abnormal cardiac calcification (heart disease)
- Calcification of soft tissue
- Easy bruising
- Eye hemorrhage
- Fractures
- Gastrointestinal bleeding
- Gum bleeding
- Heavy menstrual bleeding
- Hematuria (bloody urine)
- Hypercalciuria (calcium loss reflected in high amounts excreted in the urine)
- Osteopenia (low bone density)
- Osteoporosis (bone loss)
- Purpura (bruising associated with fragile blood vessels)
- Nosebleeds

BIRTH DEFECTS LINKED TO VITAMIN K DEFICIENCY

Because pregnant women are especially vulnerable to complications from inadequate levels of vitamin K, they must be especially attuned to making sure that their diet, medications, and lifestyle ensure optimal levels. Birth defects that have been linked to a vitamin K deficiency include the following:

- Cardiac dysfunction
- Craniofacial abnormalities
- Distal digit hyperplasia (abnormally short pinkie finger)
- Epicanthic folds (folds of the skin of the upper eyelids that partially cover the inner corner of the eyes; this is normal in Asian peoples, but not so in those of European, African, and other lineages)
- Flat nasal bridge
- Growth disorders
- Hypertelorism (excessive width between two bodily parts or organs)
- Learning disorders
- Long, thin, overlapping fingers
- Mental retardation
- Microcephaly (abnormally small head size)
- Neural tube defects
- Short nose
- Upslanting palpebral fissures (gaps between the upper and lower eyelids)

VITAMIN K_2 AND SOYBEANS

For decades, researchers have known that vitamin K_2 is composed of thirteen menaquinone forms (known as isomers), but they were not sure what roles these compounds played in the body. Gradually, scientists began experimenting with the various menaquinones, but they have only recently begun narrowing them down in terms of efficacy and their roles in the body. In Japan, for example, menaquinone-4 has been approved by the Japanese Ministry of Health as an effective therapy for treating osteoporosis. Recent studies, however, are now pointing to menaquinone-7 (MK-7) as an even more appropriate and effective therapy for osteoporosis.

Japan is one of the leading countries researching and pioneering the use of the menaquinones, and scientists there have found vitamin K_2 vital to maintaining human health. One of the primary reasons for Japan's cutting-edge interest and research is that vitamin K occurs naturally in one of Japan's staple foods—natto (fermented soybeans). Unlike other forms of fermented soybeans, such as miso and tempeh, natto is relatively unknown in the United States. Natto is made from soybeans that are washed and soaked, steamed, and then fermented with the bacterium *Bacillus natto*. It is then aged in a refrigerator.

In Japan, natto is often eaten for breakfast, sometimes mixed with rice and a raw egg or two. Natto has been a traditional Japanese food for hundreds of years, dating back to the days of ancient samurais, whose daily diet included natto because they believed it increased their strength and reaction time in battle. Ancient Japanese records point out that the leading medical professionals of the day insisted that pregnant women take a daily allowance of natto to ensure healthy offspring.

In 1980, while doing research at the University of Chicago, Dr. Hiroyuki Sumi discovered an enzyme in natto that he subsequently dubbed "nattokinase." After testing various natural ingredients and natural foods, Dr. Sumi found that the sticky threads present in natto expressed effective anti-blood-clotting abilities. When he placed natto on a blood clot, he observed that the clot

Online Information on Vitamin K

To access a U.S. Department of Agriculture list of foods ranked for vitamin K content, go online to http://www.nal.usda.gov/fnic/foodcomp/Data/SR17/wtrank/sr17w430.pdf.

To do a search for foods containing a specific nutrient, such as vitamin K, go to http://www.nal.usda.gov/fnic/foodcomp/search/ and click on "Nutrient Lists."

dissipated completely within eighteen hours. Dr. Sumi claimed that nattokinase is among the most powerful natural agents in terms of this fibrinolytic (clot-busting) activity. During the course of his research, he also discovered that vitamin K is one of the key nutrients found in natto. Today, nattokinase and its derivatives have been endorsed by the Japanese Ministry of Health as safe and beneficial, and it is now regularly recommended and prescribed by Japanese health professionals.

BEST DIETARY SOURCES OF VITAMIN K

Foods that are good sources of vitamin K include leafy vegetables, cheese, liver, and soybeans. It is also found in asparagus, coffee, bacon, and green tea.

Food	Vitamin K Content
Brussels sprouts (1/2 cup)	460 mcg
Broccoli (1/2 cup)	248 mcg
Cauliflower (1/2 cup)	150 mcg
Swiss chard (1/2 cup)	123 mcg
Spinach, uncooked (1 cup)	120 mcg
Beef (3.5 oz)	104 mcg
Pork (3.5 oz)	88 mcg
Eggs (1 whole, large)	25 mcg
Strawberries (1 cup)	23 mcg
Oats (1 oz, dry)	18 mcg
Milk, whole (8 oz)	10 mcg

Source: Northwestern University Nutrition Fact Sheet (Feinberg School) http://www.feinberg.northwestern.edu/nutrition/factsheets/vitamin-k.html

Keep reading to find out how you can reap tremendous health benefits by including vitamin K in your diet and daily supplement regimen.

2

The Menaquinone-7 (MK-7) "Miracle"

Japan was the first country to approve vitamin K_2 as a treatment for osteoporosis. Now several other countries are moving in the same direction, and many pharmaceutical companies are seeking to determine which specific menaquinone has the greater efficacy in ameliorating disease. With the mounting research demonstrating the effectiveness of MK-7, some countries and pharmaceutical companies have already started the process of making MK-7 into a prescription drug for osteoporosis.

Not only has MK-7 outshone the other menaquinones as an intervention to treat disease, but it is also fast becoming widely accepted as an effective nutritional supplement. And while few supplements even come close to rivaling the efficacy of prescription drugs, MK-7 is gaining wide acceptability in both mainstream and alternative medicine as doing just that when it comes to such maladies as osteoporosis. Its scientific pedigree is growing, and it appears likely that it will join other scientifically proven nutraceutical "druglike" supplements such as SAMe (s-adenosylmethionine), which is a prescription drug in Europe for treating depression and osteoarthritis (it is prescribed more than Prozac by doctors in Italy). Although MK-7 does not yet have the extensive drug agency approval and years of patient use that SAMe does, it certainly appears to be comparable in terms of druglike efficacy. It has also captured the attention of top scientists in both the pharmaceutical and the nutraceutical industries by virtue of its safety and the significant health benefits it confers when used in small dosages. These properties enable it to be used alongside other compounds and vitamins, like daily multivitamin-multimineral formulas.

WHY MK-7 IS SO EFFECTIVE

Researchers have confirmed that MK-7 has a profoundly positive impact on human health. MK-7 has been shown in numerous studies to actually extract calcium from the blood and arteries and then "amazingly" deposit this calcium into growing or aging bones. Although it is available only as a nutritional supplement in the United States, MK-7 appears to have the potential to prevent or even reverse some forms of heart disease and, at the same time, to do the same for bone loss, without the side effects that sometimes accompany the use of pharmaceuticals to treat these ailments. Vitamin K_2 is also more effective than vitamin E in terms of its ability to "mop up" the free radicals that damage cell membranes.

MK-7 appears to have potential to prevent or even reverse some forms of heart disease and, at the same time, to do the same for bone loss, without the side effects notoriously accompanying pharmaceuticals used to treat these ailments.

In addition to the mounting research evidence of vitamin K_2's role in preventing and even reversing osteoporosis and some forms of heart disease, other lines of research indicate that vitamin K_2 can bring about significant reductions in serum cholesterol, can prevent and possibly ameliorate Alzheimer's disease, and may be effective in addressing some forms of cancer. And recent studies indicate that vitamin K_2 (and especially MK-7) is more bioavailable and effective than vitamin K_1; thus, although multivitamin manufacturers traditionally include vitamin K_1 in their products, they may better serve us by including vitamin K_2 instead.

As mentioned previously, there are thirteen menaquinones in vitamin K_2. For several years, there has been much debate over which menaquinones are the most important or effective in disease and health. Dr. Cees Vermeer of the Netherlands is one of the leading scientists in vitamin K_2 research, and through extensive investigation, he and other scientists have found MK-7 to be one of the most effective compounds for addressing various heart and bone ailments.

Unlike vitamin K_1, MK-7 is more readily and easily absorbed and utilized in our bodies. Unfortunately, MK-7 is found only in trace amounts in food. Despite this, even small amounts of MK-7 have a profound impact on health. As we age, our bodies become less efficient at assimilating and sometimes utilizing vitamins, and we also tend to become less efficient in terms of digestion, which significantly reduces our vitamin absorption. Diseases also diminish vitamin absorption and utilization and thus can interfere with our maintaining healthy levels of vitamin K. All of these are good reasons why supplementing our diet with MK-7 is a prudent measure, whether we are seeking optimal health, are taking preventive action, or need intervention to treat a problem.

Although vitamin K_1 is still important for those who might have trouble maintaining normal blood-clotting functions, MK-7 is a better choice when it comes to common "old age" maladies such as bone loss or hardening of the arteries. In fact, MK-7 was noted in one study to be three times more effective than vitamin K_1 in improving total K status in the body. This effect was detectable after just three weeks of supplementation and was most notable after six weeks. For this reason, MK-7 is oftentimes preferable to vitamin K_1.

> Many experts predict that children who get slightly higher dosages of MK-7 on a daily basis will experience a significant decrease in calcified (hardened) arteries and bone loss later in life.

MK-7 is beneficial for all ages too, with some clinicians asserting that it is probably a good idea to give it early on to children as a preventive measure. Many experts predict that children who get slightly higher dosages of MK-7 on a daily basis will experience a significant decrease in calcified (hardened) arteries and bone loss later in life, which translates to a higher-quality (if not longer) life. This is expected to become evident during the coming decades.

THE PROOF IS IN THE STUDIES

The volume of published studies supporting MK-7's utility in promoting healthy bone and blood vessels is beginning to persuade supplement users and healthcare practitioners alike to move beyond vitamin K_1 and begin using MK-7. Indeed, not only is this form of vitamin K better, but it confers health benefits that go far beyond treating blood-clotting disorders to the prevention and treatment of age-related stiffening of arteries and bone loss (osteoporosis). The following highlights a few of these studies.

In a 1998 study carried out by M. Tamatani, S. Morimoto, M. Nakajima, and colleagues, twenty-seven Japanese men, aged sixty-four to eighty-four, had the bone mineral density (BMD) of their second to fourth lumbar vertebrae measured by dual-energy x-ray absorptiometry (DXA). It was found that the degree of bone loss increased as the levels of vitamin D, albumin (a blood protein), and MK-7 decreased. In short, the less vitamin D, albumin, and MK-7 there was in the body, the greater the degree of bone loss.

The findings in the aforementioned study were underscored in a 1995 study in Japan by M. Kaneki, Y. Mizuno, T. Hosoi, and colleagues. The scientists measured blood levels of vitamin K_1 and K_2 (menaquinone-4, -7, and -8) in twenty-four elderly women with osteoporotic spinal (vertebral) fractures and in thirty-six elderly women without fractures. They found that the major forms of vitamin K present were vitamin K_1 and MK-7, and that MK-7 levels were significantly lower in women with fractures than in those without fractures. Vitamin K_1 levels were no different in the two groups. The researchers considered "the possibility that deficiency of vitamin K, particularly that of menaquinone-7, is one of the risk factors for developing osteoporosis."

When the ovaries are removed (ovariectomy) from female rats, the rats lose hormones that protect bone integrity. In one telltale 1999 study by M. Yamaguchi, H. Taguchi, Y. H. Gao, and colleagues, rats given ovariectomies were fed a diet rich in MK-4 and MK-7. It was found that MK-7, and not MK-4, prevented loss of bone.

In a 2001 experiment by M. Yamaguchi and Z. J. Ma, bone marrow cells from the long bones (femurs) in rat legs were cultured in laboratory dishes. The bone-eroding compound parathyroid hormone or prostaglandin E2 (PGE2) was then added; both resulted in increased activity of bone-demolition cells called osteoclasts. When MK-7 was added, the bone-eroding activity of the osteoclasts was inhibited.

In a 2001 study by M. Yamaguchi, E. Sugimoto, and S. Hachiya, bone tissue from young male rats was cultured (grown) both with and without MK-7. The researchers found that bone-building compounds and the bone-forming activity of osteoblasts all increased significantly in the presence of MK-7.

In a 2002 study, M. Yamaguchi, S. Uchiyama, and Y. Tsukamato showed that when bone tissue from both young and elderly female rats was placed in laboratory dishes and cultured, the bone-forming compounds calcium, alkaline phosphatase, and deoxyribonucleic acid (DNA) were significantly decreased in the tissue from the old rats as compared with that of the young ones. MK-7 caused a significant increase in these bone-forming compounds. When the weakly estrogen-like compound genistein (from soy) was added to MK-7, the pool of available calcium for bone formation increased substantially. The researchers concluded that MK-7 "may have a preventive role for bone deterioration with aging."

In a 2003 study by M. Yamaguchi, S. Uchiyama, and Y. Tsukamato, bone tissue from aged female rats was placed in laboratory dishes to which were added factors that encourage bone breakdown (resorption), such as parathyroid hormone and PGE2. MK-7 helped inhibit this breakdown.

In a 2004 study involving elderly female rats, Y. Tsukamoto found that bone-formation players such as calcium content, alkaline phosphatase activity, and deoxyribonucleic acid (DNA) in specific bone tissues were significantly decreased compared with levels in young rats. In addition, bone-eroding compounds such as parathyroid hormone and hormonelike PGE2 caused a significant decrease in calcium content in the same bone tissues. MK-7 was found to prevent drops in the bone-forming compounds and to inhibit the activity of the bone-eroding compounds.

HOW MUCH VITAMIN K_2 IS NEEDED?

In light of what is known by scientists and what is conjectured based on solid principles of physiology, it is important to consider supplementing with vitamin K_2, and especially MK-7, in consultation with a primary healthcare practitioner. You may also want to incorporate more soy natto into your diet. Many Asian markets and grocery stores routinely stock fresh natto; some supermarket chains do too. And natto can be ordered online from companies such as the Asian Food Grocer (www.asianfoodgrocer.com).*

The official daily value (DV; once known as recommended dietary allowance, or RDA) of vitamin K is about 1 microgram (mcg) per kilogram (2.2 pounds) of body weight. However, many scientists feel this level is too low. In the body, vitamin K helps ensure that a protein called matrix Gla protein (MGP), which is found in bone, cartilage, and soft tissue, is properly processed in the body (a process called carboxylation). When this protein is undercarboxylated, these soft tissues are at risk of calcification. Although high levels of vitamin K appear to protect against this,

The authors and publisher have no financial or other interest in this company or any others mentioned in this book.

the DV errs on the low side. This has often proven to be the case in the past with other nutrients as well.

At present, the published studies have yet to fully reveal an optimum dose for vitamin K, although many experts feel 1,000–5,000 mcg (1–5 mg) would be about right. This intake lines up well with what has been found to be that of Japanese women who consume the K_2-rich fermented-soybean natto along with dark-green vegetables. A daily intake of this much vitamin K can be achieved by eating a diet rich in leafy green vegetables and fermented soy foods such as natto, and by using oral supplements rich in the main heart-healthy member of the K family, MK-7.

Unlike many vitamins, such as A and D, which are toxic in large doses, vitamin K_1 (phylloquinone) produces no toxicity, even when taken at levels five hundred times the DV for extended periods of time. As for vitamin K_2, no one yet knows for sure how much is too much or at what point taking high doses becomes wasteful or unnecessary. (On the other hand, synthetic vitamin K_3, or menadione, is known to have caused toxicity in infants given it in injectible form.)

It is likely that MK-7 should be included in everyone's daily supplementation regimen, even more so than vitamin K_1. A good daily supplemental dosage of MK-7 appears to be approximately 25–50 mcg per day, but as little as 10 mcg per day also appears to be effective. MK-7 has a seventy-two-hour half-life, meaning that the quantity taken on a Monday morning will have been used up by Thursday morning. Therefore, if a person consumes 25 mcg per day, in three days his or her body will be sporting approximately 75 mcg or more at any given time, providing daily intake is not interrupted or otherwise compromised.

SAFETY ISSUES AND ADVERSE REACTIONS WITH VITAMIN K

Intravenous (IV) administration of vitamin K_1 has produced flushing, shortness of breath (dyspnea), chest pain, cardiovascular collapse, and (rarely) death. These reactions may have been due to the vitamin itself or to agents used to disperse and emulsify the preparation. In any case, these reactions are very rare and are associated only with IV therapies.

There are few adverse effects reported for oral supplementation of vitamin K. However, menadione (vitamin K_3) is irritating to the skin and respiratory tract, and its derivatives have been implicated in producing hemolytic anemia (destruction of red blood cells), hyperbilirubinemia (excess production of the bile pigment bilirubin), and kernicterus (a jaundice condition) in newborns and especially premature infants. Menadione can also induce red-blood-cell breakdown (hemolysis) in people who are genetically deficient in an enzyme called glucose-6-phosphate dyhydrogenase. For people with severe liver disease, administration of large doses of menadione or phylloquinone (vitamin K_1) may further depress function of the organ.

Vitamin K_4 has also been linked with gastrointestinal irritation. Additionally, it has been associated with rare cases of hemolytic anemia (that is, the destruction and severe drop in numbers of red blood cells) and thrombocytopenia (low blood-platelet count) in babies. These cases typically occur in individuals with other predisposing conditions. Contact dermatitis has been found in occupational exposure to vitamins K_3 and K_4.

Oral vitamin K taken during pregnancy is most likely safe when the recommended daily value (DV) is taken. However, large dosages of vitamin K, especially K_4, given to mothers near term are associated with liver and skin conditions (hyperbilirubinemia and kernicterus) in newborns. Oral use of vitamin K during nursing appears to be very safe; however, there is insufficient data concerning the effects of high doses.

Vitamin K_3 is no longer used therapeutically because it has been linked to liver toxicity. Vitamin K_4, whether as tablets or injections, is no longer sold in the United States. Vitamin K_1, on the other hand, whether used orally, through injection, or intravenously, has been shown to be very safe in both adults and children. It has also jumped all the hurdles that are part of the Food and Drug Administration's rigorous drug approval process. Vitamin K_2 likewise appears to be safe, although additional testing is warranted. Menaquinone-4, for example, is used in Japan for treating a bone-eroding condition called osteoporotic osteopenia with no serious side effects. Menaquinone-7 appears to be safe and nontoxic even at very high doses.

Menaquinone-7 (MK-7) appears to be safe and nontoxic even at very high doses.

DRUG AND SUPPLEMENT INTERACTIONS WITH K VITAMINS

It is very important to use caution if you are taking other drugs, especially coumarins, while taking high concentrations of MK-7, whether blended in other products such as multivitamins or in its own K_2 formula. Unlike vitamin K_1, which does not accumulate in the body, MK-7 has a three-day half-life and will build up in the blood over time, establishing higher average concentrations. Unfortunately, there has been virtually no comprehensive drug interaction research on MK-7, and thus caution should be observed when taking this product in combination with other drugs. On the other hand, the beauty of MK-7 is its apparent effectiveness even at very small dosages (as little as 10 micrograms).

One group of drugs in particular called coumarins interact with vitamin K and most likely even more so with MK-7 because of its higher bioavailability. Coumarins are anticoagulants, meaning that they prevent blood-clot formation, and they are antagonists (opposing the action) of vitamin K. In one recent study, twelve subjects on anticoagulant drugs received increasing daily doses of K_1 during one-week periods. After a two-week washout, they received MK-7 on the same schedule. The conclusion was that MK-7 was approximately three to four times more potent than vitamin K_1 in interfering with coumarins or anticoagulants. Therefore, MK-7 supplementation should be decreased and used with caution by people who take coumarins or are undergoing anticoagulant therapy. (This study also demonstrated that MK-7 is superior in bioavailability and utilization to vitamin K_1.)

A very popular nutritional supplement called coenzyme Q_{10} (coQ_{10}) is chemically similar to vitamin K_2 and may have similar effects in the body. For this reason, taking coQ_{10} with vitamin K_2 may increase the risk of clotting in people taking anticoagulant drugs.

Similarly, taking herbs that are naturally rich in vitamin K, or herbs that are concentrated and thus may contain high amounts of vitamin K, could increase the risk of clotting in people taking anticoagulants. Some of these products include alfalfa, cabbage, parsley, nettle, and plantain.

Antibiotics kill off bad bacteria as well as beneficial intestinal bacteria, some of which produce vitamin K. Vitamin E at higher dosages can antagonize the effects of vitamin K and appears to reduce vitamin K absorption and inhibit K-dependent enzymes. Mineral oil also reduces gastrointestinal absorption of vitamin K and, thus, prolonged use of it is not recommended. Cholestipol (Colestid) and cholestyramine (Questran) may reduce vitamin K absorption and blood serum levels. Lastly, orlistat (Xenical) can reduce absorption. One way to offset the negative impact of orlistat is to take vitamin K at least two hours before taking the drug.

Also be aware that vitamin K levels can skew certain laboratory tests. For example, vitamin K at levels above normal can cause the liver to churn out more bilirubin and thus alter test results in babies or seniors with glucose-6-phosphate dehydrogenase (G6PD) deficiency (a hereditary condition in which red blood cells fall in number after exposure to the stress of infections or certain drugs).

Vitamin K can decrease red blood cell levels and thus alter the results of tests for red blood cell counts. Vitamin K_4 may decrease hematocrit (blood count) and blood hemoglobin levels; it also can decrease white blood cell (leukocyte) and platelet levels due to its tendency to induce a condition called pancytopenia. Vitamin K supplementation may also decrease a key compound linked to collagen formation and breakdown called hydroxyproline, which will show up in urine tests. And vitamin K supplementation can increase bone-building osteocalcin levels in postmenopausal women, increase porphyrin levels, or decrease prothrombin time (clotting time) due to its coagulation-promoting effects. Vitamin K supplementation may increase urobilinogen levels in the urine due to its ability to bring about red blood cell die-off (hemolytic anemia) in those with a G6PD enzyme deficiency. Supplementation of vitamin K can also increase protein levels, which will also show up in urine tests.

Keep in mind that although vitamin K supplementation may alter laboratory test results, it is still beneficial to your health—as long as healthcare providers are aware of it before they order specific urine and blood tests. Normally, they will ask you to discon-

Health Precautions with Vitamin K

Vitamin K should be used with caution if you have any of the following conditions or are undergoing an indicated treatment:

- Biliary fistula or obstructive jaundice
- Hemodialysis: excessive vitamin K has been linked with soft-tissue calcification
- Liver disease: vitamin K supplementation should be discontinued
- Hypoprothrombinemia: patients who don't respond to initial vitamin K therapy should discontinue it
- Reduced bile secretion: people with this condition may want to supplement with bile salts to ensure vitamin K absorption

tinue vitamin K supplementation for a week or two before these types of tests are done.

GETTING THE REAL MK-7

In most instances, it is wise to pay attention to companies and health experts who specialize or focus in specific areas, because companies that try to be "all things to all people" may not necessarily offer the best products or advice.

In the United States, there are no specific regulations or enforced testing requirements that would force manufacturers of dietary supplements to accurately reveal the quantities of the active components (called isomers) in their products. As a result, many supplement companies are taking advantage of consumers by selling supplements that contain ineffective compounds. A good example of this can be seen with SAMe. Because of the lack of regulation in the nutritional supplement industry, SAMe (s-adenosylmethionine) is so labeled that there is no way of telling how much real or "active" ingredient is in a given product. SAMe is a "natural" compound that enjoys prescription drug status in some European countries and is routinely prescribed to treat arthritis and depression. Because it occurs naturally in our bodies, it is classified as a natural product in the United States. Here, a number of companies are profiting from selling cheaply produced SAMe that contains hardly enough active ingredient to generate any benefit at all.

One potential way in which companies can mislead consumers is in promoting nontherapeutic dosages of SAMe. Although there have been at least 103 reputable double-blind, placebo studies worldwide that included more than 20,000 people and irrefutably confirmed the efficacy of this supplement, the study dosages ranged from 800–1,600 mg per day for osteoarthritis and from 1,600–3,200 mg for clinical depression. Therefore, companies recommending 200 mg per day, or even 400 mg per day, are not being fair to consumers—and especially so if they don't list the actual amount of active ingredient in their product.

Lastly, let's say two people go to different stores to purchase a SAMe product. Both labels claim to have equal amounts of SAMe, 200 mg per tablet. However, since tests for SAMe content in the United States do not distinguish between active and inactive forms (isomers) and simply lump them all together, one of these consumers may actually pay more for much less of the "real McCoy." (Inactive isomers are not toxic, but they are useless therapeutically.) Due to a lack of standardization—manufacturers are not required to quantify the amount of active isomers in their products—consumers have no way of telling the difference between high-quality and poor-quality supplements.

MK-7 is similar to SAMe in that it also contains active and inactive isomers. Many companies may be selling less-effective menaquinones rather than MK-7, or they may claim that their product contains MK-7 when it actually contains MK-4 or something else. If pure MK-7 were available today, it would cost over a half million dollars for just 1 kilogram (2.2 pounds). It is extremely difficult to produce in pure form, and up until now, no company has mastered the science of making a pure MK-7 for commercial purposes.

Here in the United States, profit often reigns supreme, and thus products that are worthless or of little efficacy abound. This undermines people's health and confuses them, and thus erodes consumer confidence in the long run. The natural products industry rakes in more than $50 billion per year. When we take into account all the companies selling ineffective or partially effective supplements, this surely amounts to billions of dollars of ineffective products being sold.

However, consumers can help offset this trend by becoming more proactive, putting in more time investigating products they want to purchase and also speaking out for proper disclosure on product labels, especially in terms of active versus inactive ingredients. They can begin by writing product manufacturers for verification of product content, especially with reference to the milligrams or international units (IU) of the active ingredients or chemical components present.

With regard to menaquinone-7, although a product label may state "Vitamin K_2 with MK-7," this is misleading, as all vitamin K_2 has MK-1 through MK-13. What labels need to reveal is the *exact amount* of MK-7 in the product, with a goal of using this disclosure to help ensure consumers a daily intake of least 25 micrograms (mcg) per day of MK-7.

Another misleading claim states that only natto-based products contain the best source of MK-7. This is simply not true. As mentioned above, consumers need to know the exact amount of MK-7 they are getting in a daily dose of supplements. Even Dr. Sumi, the discoverer of nattokinase, points out that there are several other well-known starting materials that contain MK-7. Some of these include black beans, adzuki beans, kidney beans, and sunflower seeds.

The bottom line is that consumers must insist on knowing how much active MK-7 there is in any vitamin K product and then take enough to get at least 25 mcg per day.

3

Vitamin K_2 and Other Therapies for a Healthy Heart

Heart disease, cancer, and diabetes number among the top ten killers of adult Americans and, in many instances, appear to be linked to or influenced by dietary and lifestyle factors. Of course, living and the passage of time exacts a toll on us all. Other animals share this vulnerability: sharks, rats, humans, and other species get cancer, and there is even fossil evidence of arthritis-like conditions and tumors in some dinosaurs. But by and large, most nonhuman mammals are spared high blood pressure, heart disease, diabetes, obesity, and similar conditions collectively referred to as "the diseases of civilization."

Why? Is it because they do not live as long as humans? Not necessarily, as some species are relatively long-lived: tortoises can live nearly two hundred years, as do some fish. But they are not genetically close to us. What of our evolutionary cousins and siblings? In the wild, chimpanzees live, on average, about thirty-five to forty years. This life span matched or exceeded that of our forebears for countless millennia, but it has been surpassed by humans during the past sixty years or so. This, most scientists concede, is attributable to improved nutrition and disease prevention and treatment. So, it would seem that we are doing better than our evolutionary relatives on the whole. But are we really?

Let's turn this question around. Do hypertension, heart disease, and other chronic conditions appear in chimpanzees who reach middle age and advanced age? While some diseases such as

HEART TRIVIA: DID YOU KNOW?

- The existence of the heart was well known to the Greeks, who gave it the name *kardia,* which has endured in English as *cardiac.* The great philosopher-scientist Aristotle believed that the heart was the seat of the soul.
- Most people believe that their heart is on the left side of their chest, but this is not true. The heart is actually located almost in the center of the chest, between the lungs.
- The average heart beats 72 times per minute, which comes to over 100,000 times a day and 38 million times or so in one year. By the time a man or woman reaches age seventy, his or her heart will have beaten 2.5 billion times.
- The largest artery in the body, the aorta, has almost the same diameter as a common garden hose. The smallest blood vessels in the human body are the capillaries—it takes ten of them to equal the thickness of a single human hair
- The human body has about 6 quarts (5.6 liters) of blood circulating in it. In a single day, this volume of blood travels a total of 12,000 miles (19,000 km).
- The heart pumps about 48 million gallons of blood during an average lifetime, enough to fill three supertankers and then some!
- As we get older, maximum heart rate decreases.

cancer do occur in aging chimps, the rates appear to be far lower than one would expect if the aging process alone were the culprit. All things considered, the "diseases of civilization" such as heart disease occur at remarkably low rates in our aged evolutionary relatives. The "why" behind this health discrepancy between chimps and humans may hold the key to our collective quest for maximal health and longevity.

In chimps and other nonhuman animals, diet and physical activity patterns are basically in harmony with the evolved nature of each species. For example, chimpanzees eat and engage in patterns of physical exertion that are consistent with very ancient and entrenched patterns. Humans, on the other hand, have deviated greatly from the dietary and health-conducive physical activity that characterized our branch of the primate family tree for hundreds of thousands of years.

During the course of the past forty years or so, evidence has steadily accrued indicating that humans achieve and maintain optimal health on a diet that consists largely of protein, specific complex carbohydrates, and certain fats. Indeed, the dietary pattern that anthropologists and various nutrition experts have found to be most consonant with our evolved nature is one referred to as the Paleolithic or "Old Stone Age" diet. It is one few people in the West follow today. And it is this mismatch between our ancient metabolic machinery and relatively recent dietary patterns—patterns that arose during the past ten thousand years (Neolithic or "New Stone Age" to present)—that many experts feel underlies the rise of chronic diseases such as heart disease.

But aren't we living longer and healthier? At the turn of the last century, the average American woman could expect to live to be about fifty-one years of age. The average man could expect to blow out at least forty-eight candles on his birthday cake before being visited by the Grim Reaper. By 1998, these averages had grown considerably: women can now expect to live to be eighty years old and men seventy-four years old. According to public health sources, these gains in the American life span are the result, *at least in part,* of reductions in infant mortality, infectious diseases among infants and children, and such basic public health measures as safer drinking water, widespread vaccination programs, better nutrition, and an improved standard of living. Other factors include improved screening and treatment of certain cancers, declines in tobacco use among adults, and improvements in the medical management of many chronic diseases.

We are indisputably living longer, but there is plenty of room for improvement. Americans are generally overweight and out of shape. Researchers have linked obesity and a lack of exercise to the development of heart disease and high blood pressure. Today, heart disease and stroke are leading causes of death among adults in the United States. These are "diseases of civilization"—diseases whose development and course are, many scientists tell us, slowed or otherwise beneficially impacted by dietary, nutritional, and exercise factors. And vitamin K_2 can be one of these factors, making a significant contribution to a heart-friendly lifestyle.

Heart disease and stroke are "diseases of civilization"—diseases whose development and course are, many scientists tell us, slowed or otherwise beneficially impacted by dietary, nutritional, and exercise factors. And vitamin K_2 can be one of these factors, making a significant contribution to a heart-friendly lifestyle.

THE MECHANICS OF CHANGE

This brings us to the question of the mechanics of change. We read almost daily newspaper articles on the health benefits of specific foods, beverages, fitness pursuits, and so on. And yet, swimming in information though we are, only about 3 percent of Americans actually act on what they know. Is this attributable to laziness, information overload, or both? Or maybe it is that other concerns crowd out doing what we know is best—grabbing a burger at a corner fast-food place makes it possible to eat and get back to work in thirty minutes. Perhaps we have just come to expect instant answers in what has become an age of instant foods, instant online access to information, and instant gratification. Then, too, we are by and large inveterate gamblers insofar as we have a tendency to think the person down the street will not get away with his or her unhealthy lifestyle choices, but we will.

If you stop for a moment and think in terms of your own life, you probably will see many of these factors at work. Human nature being what it is, most of us prefer convenience, speed, and comfort over working at staying well and fit. In light of this, we need to zero in on relatively easy-to-make changes that will help us maximize our health and quality of life. Even simple changes can confer rich heart-friendly dividends.

CAUSES OF HEART DISEASE

While all the causes and players in the development of arterial blockage are not yet fully identified and explored, many have been. Among them are the following.

- Systemic (whole body) inflammation
- Failure to "mop up" cell-damaging compounds, especially those that damage arterial walls, such as homocysteine and free radicals (homocysteine is a sulfur-containing amino acid that is produced during normal metabolic activity in the body and that, in high enough amounts, contributes to the development of cardiovascular disease; free radicals are highly reactive chemicals that can damage, by oxidation, other molecules)
- An overabundance of blood vessel–clogging oxidized low-density lipoprotein (LDL) cholesterol combined with average or low levels of high-density lipoprotein (HDL) cholesterol, which shuttles bad cholesterol from blood vessels back to the liver
- High blood pressure
- Diabetes
- Obesity and lack of exercise
- Familial tendencies to develop blood vessel diseases
- A diet high in saturated fats, which clog arteries and generate free radicals, or an imbalanced intake of fats that protect blood vessels; that is, too high an intake of omega-6 fatty acids, such as are found in corn oil, and too little consumption of omega-3 fatty acid foods, such as are found in many types of fish and walnuts

- Inadequate consumption of compounds that protect blood vessels, such as resveratrol (found in grapes and red wine), certain B vitamins such as folic acid, s-adenosylmethionine (SAMe), vitamin C, and vitamin E

BLOOD VISCOSITY AND ARTERIAL DISEASE

One of the ways in which all these negatives tend to cause heart disease is by making blood viscous or thick. Blood that is viscous tends to create friction on blood vessels, especially in areas of turbulent blood flow such as where vessels fork and go in two different directions. When blood is viscous (think of thick ketchup or sludge), it damages blood vessel walls. The cells that line damaged arteries and veins will attempt to adapt to the assault and offset the impact by building up plaque.

The damage done to the artery walls causes the body to send in macrophages, cells that devour foreign material in the body as well as dead and dying cells. When these macrophages increase their numbers and at the same time take in "bad" cholesterol (oxidized LDL), they become what are called foam cells. These foam cells create fatty streaks that are the first stages of atherosclerosis (blockage in blood vessels). As this process continues, a fibrous mass builds up, a mass filled with lipids (fats) and calcium that's called an atheroma.

At this point, coronary artery disease is well underway. And as the blockage or plaque builds, blood pressure can rise precipitously. If an atheroma should rupture and release a clot that travels and blocks a major blood vessel feeding the heart, a myocardial infarction (heart attack) occurs. If the clot blocks a vessel that feeds the brain, a stroke takes place.

If you smoke, have high blood pressure, are diabetic, drink excessively, do drugs, have a high homocysteine level, or have any of the other factors discussed above, then your blood viscosity increases, as does your risk of developing significant blockage in circulatory vessels that get the brunt of the movement ("shear stress") of this sticky, viscous blood. Since heart disease is the number-one killer of adult Americans, it follows that a lot of us are walking around with this sludge in our circulatory systems.

REDUCING YOUR RISK OF HEART DISEASE

Here are some of the things you can do to lower the risk of getting heart disease:

- If you smoke, stop.
- If you drink alcohol excessively, curtail your intake or stop.
- If you use recreational drugs, stop doing so and look into therapies to help your body repair any existing multiorgan damage.
- Take a full-spectrum or complete B multiple vitamin. This will help the body deal with arterial wall–damaging homocysteine.
- Take an antioxidant supplement. Antioxidants help the body deal with the cell-damaging free radicals generated by viscous blood.
- If you are obese, get the excess weight off slowly under medical supervision. The "Paleodiet" is highly recommended (check out the Paleodiet at http://14ushop.com/wizard/living-longer.html).
- Eat foods low in saturated fat. Favor foods that are rich in omega-3 fatty acids, such as cold-water fish species (for example, salmon and tuna), over those high in omega-6 fatty acids, such as cereals, eggs, poultry, most vegetable oils, baked goods, and margarine.
- If you are diabetic, keep your condition under control and ask your doctor about the use of L-carnosine (beta-alanyl-L-histidine, a marriage of the amino acids beta-alanine and histidine), the drug aminoguanidine, and acetyl-L-carnitine, all of which prevent sugars from interacting with free amino acids in such a way as to generate tissue-damaging compounds referred to as

advanced glycation end products (AGEs). And inquire about other factors that help counter the cellular and tissue damage caused by high and fluctuating blood sugar levels, such as R-lipoic acid and bilberry extract.

- If your LDL ("bad") cholesterol level is high, work with your doctor or dietitian to reduce it.
- If your triglyceride (storage fats) or fibrinogen (a protein involved in coagulation) level is high, ask your healthcare provider about niacin or other approaches for reducing it.
- Clean up dental infections and inflammation in the body. Make sure your healthcare practitioner monitors your C-reactive protein level, as this protein goes up in concert with inflammation.
- If you are stressed out or depressed, consider stress-management courses or cognitive therapy.
- Consume lots of brown-algae foods such as wakame and kombu. These algae contain compounds called fucoidans that may act as mild blood thinners, reducing blood viscosity.
- If you have high blood pressure, make sure to take the medications your doctor prescribes. If you have mild hypertension, ask your doctor about ways to reduce it using diet, exercise, and perhaps nonpharmaceutical compounds, such as celery seed extract, potassium, and the mild herbal diuretic corn silk (*Zea mays*), that complement traditional approaches.
- If you have arterial or peripheral blockage already, ask your doctor about dietary approaches to reversing it, such as Dr. Dean Ornish's very low-fat dietary program.

THE ROLE OF VITAMIN K

People who develop atherosclerosis often are found to have calcification present in their arteries, something more commonly known as "hardening of the arteries." Interestingly, there are some links between the process that hardens arteries and that which keeps bones hard. One of these links lies with the activity of the vitamin K family.

In bones, vitamin K (K_1 and K_2) plays a role in the production of the proteins osteocalcin and matrix Gla protein (MGP). Both contribute to the genesis of bone and its integrity. Both also must undergo carboxylation before they become effective in bone formation. Carboxylation is the melding of a carboxyl group (-COOH) or carbon dioxide with a compound. Vitamin K acts as a cofactor that facilitates the carboxylation of osteocalcin and MGP.

As it turns out, MGP not only is a contributor to bone matrix formation but also is a potent inhibitor of calcification of arteries and cartilage. There is, in fact, evidence that when vitamin K levels fall below certain levels, MGP is not generated in sufficient quantities to prevent arterial calcification. In laboratory studies, mice who fail to produce enough MGP develop extensive calcification of their blood vessels. Humans, too, appear to suffer in a similar way when vitamin K levels are too low.

Support for this idea comes from research done in the Netherlands. As part of a study to assess the role of vitamin K levels in atherosclerosis, scientists gleaned data from the Rotterdam Study. This particular study was started in 1990 in Ommoord, a suburb of Rotterdam, and involved tracking 10,994 men and women aged fifty-five and over. The purpose of the study was to investigate the prevalence, incidence, and risk factors for various chronic diseases in the elderly, including cardiovascular, neurologic, movement, and various eye diseases. This vitamin K–atherosclerosis study focused on analyzing dietary data on 4,807 participants with no history of heart attack, tracking them until the year 2000.

Researchers found that both vitamin K_1 (phylloquinone) and vitamin K_2 were associated with artery-beneficial high-density lipoproteins (HDL), and vitamin K_2 caused a decrease in total cholesterol. Compared with those whose vitamin K_2 intake was in the lowest third of the participants, those whose intake was in the top third boasted a 41 percent reduction in both fatal and nonfatal heart attacks, sudden cardiac death, and other forms of heart disease related to compromised arterial blood flow. In addition, death from both coronary heart disease and all other causes was significantly reduced for those with the highest vitamin K levels. Most intriguing of all was the fact that participants who had a high vitamin K_2 intake had the lowest levels of calcification in their aortas, while low vitamin K intake was linked to an increased risk of death from coronary heart disease.

Most intriguing of all was the fact that participants who had a high vitamin K_2 intake had the lowest levels of calcification in their aortas, while low vitamin K intake was linked to an increased risk of death from coronary heart disease.

THE "STONE AGE" DIET AND HEART DISEASE

When it comes to vitamin K_2, our Stone Age ancestors had a great advantage over us in two primary ways. For one, they ate only natural and mostly raw foods, which insured a higher nutrient value compared with the processed foods that are so prevalent in today's Western diet. Second, our ancestors' diet was virtually free of chemicals, antibiotics, and drugs that destroy the beneficial intestinal bacteria that produce vitamin K. However, when it comes to a heart-healthy diet, there's a lot more to consider:

The Western diet and lifestyle by and large contain too much of the kinds of things that foster the development of heart disease. We chow down on foods that contain artery-damaging fats such as trans-fatty acids, too much sodium, inadequate fiber and antioxidants, and lots of calorie-rich sweets. Our taste, or even craving, for fat and sugary things is an ancient pattern wired into our brains. Our ancestors needed energy to stay healthy and survive. Fats and sugars are to us what long-lasting batteries are to a certain perpetual-motion bunny on TV.

We are, according to many anthropologists, modern folk running about with "Stone Age" brains. We are adapted to seek out fatty foods and sweet stuff, resulting in a deep-seated craving that isn't easily surmounted or tamed. And perhaps it shouldn't be. In a study carried out on the tropical island of Kitava in Papua New Guinea, field researchers surveyed 2,300 native islanders aged twenty to ninety-six with respect to heart disease patterns and found that these so-called primitive people got a lot of their daily calories from fat. Most surprisingly, these scientists found that sudden cardiac death and stroke were extremely rare in Kitavans. All the adults surveyed were relatively thin and had blood pressure readings lower than that of the average Westerner. Interestingly, the Kitavans' serum cholesterol was a little high, probably due to their high intake of saturated fat from coconuts.

The diet of the Kitavans was mainly tubers, fruit, fish, and coconuts. They consumed little Western food or alcohol. Saturated fat intake from coconut was high, as was their intake of omega-3 polyunsaturated fatty acids, soluble fiber, and minerals. Salt intake was quite low compared with levels in the West. As for physical activity, the Kitavans were found to be slightly more physically active than sedentary Western populations. However, *80 percent of both sexes were daily smokers.*

Other published research underscores what was seen in the Kitavans. So, does fat play a role in the genesis of heart disease or not? Does it help turn blood into thick corn syrup and thus damage arteries or not? Here we have a population of people eating a lot of fat, smoking, and being only slightly more active than Westerners, and they are thinner, have a lower average resting blood pressure than most of us, and have virtually no heart disease. What's protecting the Kitavans? What are they doing that we in the United States are not?

While there is no clear consensus among scientists, there is sufficient evidence to indicate that the *kind* of fats consumed is a key player in the development of heart disease. Westerners eat too much of the artery-clogging fats like trans-fatty acids (the "bad" fat in stick margarine, for example) as well as saturated fats.

But wait a minute: the Kitavans eat *lots* of saturated fat, have higher serum cholesterol levels than most Westerners, and yet have almost no cardiovascular disease. Why? The verdict isn't in, but the protective factor appears to be the high levels of omega-3 fatty acids in the "Stone Age" diet of the Kitavans. Omega-3 fatty acids are the main fats in cold-water fish and have been shown to protect against the development of blood vessel blockage.

So why isn't the Kitavans' smoking wreaking havoc in their arteries? Again, the answer appears to lie in the amounts of omega-3-rich foods the Kitavans consume daily. These fatty acids protect cell membranes from incurring the sort of damage that appears to favor the development of heart disease and even some cancers. In Japan, where 59 percent of men smoke, lung cancer rates are lower than one would expect. Many epidemiologists and other researchers feel that the Japanese penchant for eating lots of omega-3-rich sushi, sashimi, and other foods underlies this trend. (But no, this is not to say that it is okay to smoke. Smokers who consume high levels of omega-3 fatty acids still get cancer.)

What this body of evidence suggests in terms of fleshing out a "balanced diet" that lines up with our evolved nature is this: when the daily fat bug bites, you should satisfy it with the health-protective fats. Instead of chowing down on foods rich in saturated or trans-fatty acids, make a practice of eating omega-3-rich fish, such as lake trout, tuna, and salmon, and foods rich in monounsaturated fats, such as olive, flaxseed, and peanut oils and avocados. Peanuts, walnuts, and wheat germ are also good sources of omega-3 fatty acids.

For those who cannot lay their hands on fresh fish or just happen not to favor eating fish, fish-oil capsules can be found at most health food stores and even many pharmacies. It should be noted that people with diabetes as well as people on blood thinners should first discuss using fish-oil supplements with a physician, as the supplements can exacerbate or complicate diabetes and interact badly with blood thinners.

WHAT EXACTLY IS A BALANCED DIET?

What goes into making a balanced diet, and what exactly is a balanced diet anyway? (Hint: It isn't a cream-filled pastry in each hand.) Briefly, a balanced diet is one in which you eat a varied enough intake of foods to furnish your body with the vitamins and minerals it needs to avoid deficiencies as well as to prevent certain chronic diseases, such as heart disease. Dietary needs vary according to life stage, your lifestyle, and your particular health pedigree. The experts suggest that we select foods from five major food groups each day. These are:

- Vegetables
- Fruits
- Breads, cereals, rice, and pasta
- Milk, yogurt, and cheese
- Meat, poultry, fish, beans, eggs, and nuts

Since breads, cereals, rice, pasta, beans, milk, yogurt, and cheese were introduced into the human diet during the past ten thousand years or so, some anthropologists and healthcare professionals feel that we are not really adapted to consuming them. Our metabolic machinery, if you will, is much older and is geared to thrive on a diet high in protein, low in sodium but high in potassium, and high in fruit and certain vegetables.

There is a growing body of evidence indicating that a balanced diet lies in adopting a Paleolithic or "Stone Age" diet. Proponents point to the fact that many of the more recent dietary additions, such as wheat, beans, and milk, evoke allergic reactions in many people. Milk proteins have also been implicated in the onset of juvenile diabetes.

And evidence is accruing that indicates that people who eat a so-called primitive diet—one high in protein, high in complex carbohydrates such as potassium-rich fruit, but low or devoid of beans, potatoes, rice, cereals, and milk—typically have few of the chronic diseases that plague Western societies. Interestingly, this kind of "primitive diet" is rich in the powerful antioxidant alpha-lipoic acid, as well as B vitamins that reduce elevated homocysteine levels.

All in all, while still controversial, it does make sense that a diet consistent with our evolved nature is probably going to produce more health benefits than a diet at odds with it. Recent scientific studies appear to bear this out. For example, in a fourteen-year study involving more than 80,000 women, scientists at Harvard Medical School discovered that women with the highest protein intakes were 26 percent less likely than those who ate the least protein to develop ischemic heart disease. More important, protein-rich diets benefited these women *regardless* of their fat intake.

Until a consensus emerges from all the studies, it is probably wise to minimize your intake of "non-Paleo" foods like milk, cereals, and grains and to eat a diet rich in vegetables, fruits, and foods containing high levels of omega-3 fatty acids and protein, including cold-water fish and walnuts.

FOODS AND NUTRITIONAL SUPPLEMENTS THAT BENEFIT THE HEART

There is a vast number of well-known vitamins, minerals, and dietary supplements that help support and sustain a healthy heart and circulatory system. However, when it comes to addressing the reduction and even reversal of arterial calcification with natural products, vitamin K_2—specifically MK-7—is gradually becoming accepted as one of the most effective players. Meanwhile, there are many other effective compounds that can be found in foods, such as omega-3-rich fish (salmon and tuna), garlic, walnuts, and curry. Others, depending on dietary imbalances and deficiencies and

When it comes to addressing the reduction and even reversal of arterial calcification with natural products, vitamin K_2—specifically MK-7—is gradually becoming accepted as one of the most effective players.

individual lifestyle and genetic propensities, may need to be taken as supplements. Keep in mind that any supplement program needs to be discussed with and supervised by a physician, dietitian, or other qualified healthcare professional who has substantive training in dietetics, nutrition science, and drug–vitamin interactions.

Cayenne

One of the best culinary spices that can favorably influence circulatory health is cayenne, also known as hot red pepper. A number of scientific studies have found that this favorite of hot-food aficionados lowers artery-clogging cholesterol and triglycerides.

In Thailand, medical researchers took particular note of the fact that people who consume fairly large quantities of cayenne have a lower incidence of potentially dangerous blood clots (thromboembolisms). Intrigued, the scientists surveyed medical records of people in countries where hot and spicy foods are regularly consumed and found that folks who eat a lot of cayenne in their diet have a much lower incidence of blood-clotting diseases.

This is logical given the fact that cayenne contains compounds that have fibrinolytic activity, meaning that they are able to break up blood clots. And working cayenne into your diet is, of course, relatively easy to do. Foods can readily be seasoned with cayenne powder and sauce. Supermarkets carry plenty of foods laced with hot red pepper, and it is fairly easy to locate Asian and Mexican restaurants in most metropolitan cities throughout the world.

Garlic

Garlic may also help fight arterial blockage in many ways. Various studies have found that garlic protects against free radicals, reduces the tendency of the blood to clot, and possibly lowers both blood pressure and cholesterol levels. In at least one published study, garlic was found to raise levels of the artery-protective high-density lipoproteins (HDL). Garlic can be used fresh by adding it to foods, or it can be taken as a supplement.

Turmeric

The yellow spice turmeric, used in curry dishes, has shown effectiveness in lowering cholesterol. It also combats inflammation, which is implicated in the genesis of arterial blockage (as well as various cancers, Alzheimer's disease, and a host of other human afflictions). Turmeric can easily be added to foods as a spice or taken as a supplement.

Tea

Tea helps disarm some of the players that contribute to heart disease. Black, white, and green teas contain compounds called polyphenols, which lower cholesterol and triglyceride levels, as well as flavonoids, which prevent the artery-blocking low-density lipoprotein (LDL) cholesterol from undergoing significant oxidation. (If you are not acquainted with oxidation, leave a pat of butter out at room temperature for a few weeks. It will go rancid due to the oxidation process.)

In 1989, coauthor Dr. Payne carried out a pilot study to gauge the effects of a Chinese black tea variety called Yunnan Tuocha on patients with high serum cholesterol levels. A group of these patients drank one cup of the tea with meals but did not otherwise change their diet or lifestyle. These patients were compared with a matched group that did not drink the tea or make any other changes to their diet or lifestyle. Those in the "tea tipping" group who consistently drank the tea experienced an average drop in total cholesterol of 19.3 percent after thirty days, while those who belonged to the "tea-less" group experienced no significant decline in their cholesterol level.

The addition of green, white, or black tea to the diet is relatively easy and inexpensive. However, people who take monoamine oxidase inhibitors (MAOIs) should take note: the caffeine in these teas could cause problems. Also, those taking a blood-thinning drug such as warfarin should not drink large amounts of tea, green especially; green tea contains vitamin K, which will directly counteract the drug's blood-thinning action. Keep in mind, however, that vitamin K_2 and especially MK-7 combined with some of these natural ingredients create a very effective and synergistic natural regimen.

Omega-3 Fatty Acids

According to the American Heart Association (AHA), epidemiological and clinical trials have shown that omega-3 fatty acids reduce the risk of cardiovascular disease. People with high triglyceride levels and patients with cardiovascular disease should talk to their doctor about taking omega-3 supplements to help stem progression. Omega-3 fatty acids can be obtained in the diet from fish and plant sources. The AHA recommends eating fish (particularly fatty fish) at least two times a week. Fatty fish like mackerel, lake trout, herring, sardines, albacore tuna, and salmon are high in the omega-3 fatty acids eicosapentaenoic acid (EPA) and docosahexaenoic acid (DHA). The AHA also recommends eating tofu and other forms of soybeans, canola, walnuts, and flaxseed, and their oils, which contain alpha-linolenic acid (LNA), which the body converts to omega-3 fatty acids.

Coenzyme Q_{10} (CoQ_{10})

CoQ_{10}, also called ubiquinone, is produced throughout the human body and plays a role in many body processes, especially in the energy-producing machinery of each cell, the mitochondria. Large amounts are manufactured in the liver and are then utilized readily by the heart, an organ heavily dependent on the oxidative energy produced by mitochondria. According to some studies,

Supplements for Homocysteine Management

Homocysteine is an amino acid produced in our bodies and found in the blood that appears to irritate blood vessels and increase blood-clotting tendencies, which can increase the risk for heart disease, stroke, and vascular disease. Normally, the body converts homocysteine into the sulfur-rich amino acid methionine, which is utilized to build proteins, but this process requires an adequate intake of folic acid and vitamins B_6 and B_{12} (methylcobalamin). In addition, there are several genes involved that influence how the body uses folate and vitamins B_6 and B_{12}. When one or more of these genes is defective, it can predispose a person to folate deficiency, which leads to high levels of homocysteine. One way to ensure an adequate intake of these nutrients plus others involved in homocysteine regulation, such as s-adenosylmethionine (SAMe), is to take an oral supplement rich in all these factors.

people under age thirty produce about 300 milligrams of coQ_{10} per day, while older people and those on statins and other drugs that affect the liver tend to synthesize less. Some researchers feel that certain "old age" heart ailments like congestive heart failure may have their origin or be exacerbated by a coQ_{10} deficiency. CoQ_{10} is nontoxic even in high doses and has been found to be of benefit in preventing or ameliorating a wide range of diseases and conditions, including certain heart ailments, cancers, mitochondrial disorders, and neurodegenerative diseases, such as Parkinson's disease, Huntington's disease, and amyotrophic lateral sclerosis (ALS). This argues for supplementation in folks over age thirty.

Magnesium

Many studies have found decreased mortality from cardiovascular diseases in people who routinely consume water containing high levels of magnesium along with calcium and fluoride. One large study that tracked almost fourteen thousand men and women found that higher serum magnesium levels were associated with a decreased risk of coronary heart disease in women, though not in men. Perhaps the benefits that might have accrued in men were offset by other aspects of their lifestyle or diet. Then, too, modern populations often consume magnesium at levels way out of proportion to the level our ancestors evolved to thrive on over millions of years. For example, contemporary populations consume almost four parts of calcium to one part of magnesium, an out-of-kilter intake that actually leads to a loss of magnesium! In light of this, it would be prudent to take in at least as much magnesium as calcium on a daily basis through diet and (when needed) supplementation. For adults, 1,000–1,200 mg of calcium and an equal quantity of magnesium should ensure optimal levels of both minerals and thus help prevent certain cardiovascular diseases.

CONCLUSION

Worldwide, it is well established that heart health is a major factor in the human condition. Maintaining a healthy heart and dealing with heart and cardiovascular ailments is not simple or easy. As shown in this chapter, heart health is a packaged deal that requires an assortment of positive behaviors and healthy choices—including, but not limited to, supplementation with vitamin K_2. So, in addition to taking K_2 and following a heart-healthy diet, be sure to engage in other activities and behaviors that can help prevent, cure, or maintain the health of your heart. Also, consider the other heart-healthy supplements described in this chapter. While vitamin K_2 can do a lot for your heart health, it is only part of the solution.

■ 4 ■

Vitamin K_2 and Other Therapies for Healthy Bones

The human skeleton contains 206 bones that work together to keep us from collapsing into a puddle of limp tissues like a jellyfish out of water. They also protect our vulnerable internal organs, such as the heart, lungs, and brain. Most of us pay little attention to our bones unless we break one or experience severe bone loss (osteoporosis) or a serious bone disease. This may be a natural tendency, but it isn't particularly wise. By the time bone loss, for example, is obvious, it is more difficult to slow or reverse than would have been the case earlier in the process.

Fortunately, there are dietary steps and other ways to build strong bones and prevent or slow bone loss. To understand how these work, it helps to know a little about how bones are formed and maintained, and also what can happen to cause significant bone loss. Let's take a look.

BONE BIOLOGY 101

What do you picture when you hear the word *bone*? Probably something solid and devoid of life, like the bone a dog might chew on or the famed cattle skulls that adorn belt buckles and bolo ties throughout the southwestern United States. But bones are neither solid nor nonliving. They are, in fact, composed of tissues that are among the most active in the human body. Bone is composed of a dense outer shell that encases the trabecula or

BONE TRIVIA: DID YOU KNOW?

- We are all born with 300 bones in our bodies. However, by the time we reach adulthood, we wind up with only 206 bones. This occurs because separate bones fuse together to make a single bone.
- Adult human bones account for 14 percent of the body's total weight.
- The wrists, hands, and fingers contain a total of fifty-four bones.
- The smallest bone in the body is found in the inner ear—the stirrup bone.
- The longest bone in the body is the femur, which accounts for approximately 25 percent of a person's overall height.
- The face is made up of fourteen bones.
- A chandelier made up of human bones hangs in a small chapel in the Czech Republic.

spongy bone. When significant bone loss occurs, the "holes" in the spongy inner tissue grow larger and more numerous, weakening the bone's internal structure.

During our lifetime, bone is being continuously broken down and reabsorbed, while new bone is being created (a process referred to as bone remodeling). This remodeling cycle is essential to maintain skeletal integrity (homeostasis), to keep bones elastic, and to generate a steady source of extracellular calcium. This intricate dance between bone breakdown and bone building results in our entire skeletons being replaced every seven years.

The interplay between bone construction and demolition leans heavily toward the building side during childhood through young adulthood. During this time, most of the total bone mineral content is being deposited, a process that is virtually complete by the time most people reach their early twenties. Then, beginning at about age thirty, the balance begins to shift away from building to demolition. Bone loss begins to exceed bone formation to the tune of about 1 percent per year. In women, bone demolition cells called osteoclasts are revved up by a loss of estrogen. A subsequent elevation of inflammatory compounds stimulates the breakdown of bone in the body, and vital mineral content is transported to the blood.

Bone health thus hinges on a balance between bone building and bone breakdown. When things get out of kilter—when the interplay between them becomes disjointed or, in medical parlance, "uncoupled"—the dance between bone formation and resorption begins to favor bone loss.

Normally, bone resorption happens very quickly, which results in most of the bone remodeling activity being focused on bone formation. This building process includes the manufacture of collagen and other organic components as well as the addition of minerals to bone matrix. Among the biochemical indicators that can be measured to assess the state of bone building in the body are total alkaline phosphatase, skeletal alkaline phosphatase, procollagen-I extension peptide, and osteocalcin. Biochemical indicators that can be measured to assess the state of bone resorption are calcium, hydroxyproline, total pyridinolines, free deoxypyridinoline, N-telopeptide, and C-telopeptide. If bone resorption rates are high or normal but bone formation rates are low, bone loss (osteoporosis) begins to occur and can place sufferers at risk of bone fractures (most often involving bones in the spine, hip, and wrist) and skeletal deformity (such as women and men with a profound hump on their back called the "dowager's hump").

With repeated triggering of bone turnover, such as occurs during the postmenopausal period in women, as well as in health conditions involving the production of excess hormones (for example, parathyroid hormone, cortisol, thyroid hormone, or spreading cancer), bone formation rates shoot up but tend to lag behind resorption rates. Also, some elderly patients tend to have resorption rates that are normal and bone-building rates that are lower than normal. These biological situations represent a surefire formula for bone loss over time.

WHO IS MOST AT RISK OF DEVELOPING OSTEOPOROSIS?

Bone loss occurs when the breakdown activities outstrip the building ones. One of the risk factors for developing this out-of-kilter bodily scenario is being female. Asian and white women tend to be at greater risk than black women. Women who have a prolonged absence of menstrual periods as well as those who are postmenopausal (including menopause brought on by a hysterectomy including removal of the ovaries) also have a greater risk of developing osteoporosis. It should be pointed out, however, that 10 percent of black women over age fifty have osteoporosis, as do 24 percent of white men and 17 percent of black men eighty years of age or older.

Additional risk factors for bone loss include the following:

- Older age (starting in the mid-thirties but accelerating after fifty)
- Having a small bone structure
- Having a non-Hispanic white or Asian ethnic background
- Having a family history of osteoporosis or an osteoporosis-related fracture in a parent or sibling
- Having had a fracture following a low-level injury, especially after the age of fifty
- A history of having been sedentary or even immobile; lack of exercise
- Smoking or excessive intake of alcohol or caffeine
- Having a deficiency of a sex hormone such as estrogen; this holds true in both women (menopausal, especially) and men
- A low dietary intake and/or absorption of calcium and vitamin D

- A history of abnormal weight loss with corresponding loss of key minerals (anorexia nervosa or bulimia)
- Use of medications such as glucocorticoid drugs (for example, prednisone), excess thyroid hormone replacement, or use of the blood-thinner heparin or certain anticonvulsant medications, such as phenytoin (Dilantin) and ethotoin (Peganone)
- A history of diseases that are known to affect the integrity of

MEASURING BONE LOSS

Years ago, x-rays of bones were about the only way to assess bone loss, but this was wholly unreliable in catching early bone loss. In fact, 30 to 40 percent of bone mineral must be lost before bone loss is detectable on a routine x-ray. Thankfully, better detection technology was developed that allows doctors to bring to light even small decreases in bone mass. The most widely available and preferred technique is called dual-energy x-ray absorptiometry (DEXA).

During DEXA, a patient lies on a table while a mechanical arm passes back and forth over the body part or segment being measured. No injections or dyes are employed during this procedure, the radiation exposure is minuscule (one-sixth of that in a typical chest x-ray), and patients being tested experience no pain or discomfort. The process is quick; the x-ray beam typically maps out the amount of calcium in the bone in only about five to seven minutes. A computer then calculates the amount of bone mineral and compares it to established values for people of the same age and sex as the patient.

Newer, more cost-effective techniques such as ultrasound for screening bone mass are now becoming available. This approach, however, cannot measure bone mass at sites of osteoporotic fracture such as the hip or spine. In addition, some experts have voiced reservations about whether ultrasound can accurately measure bone mass, although the results of recent studies indicate that ultrasound is indeed an effective tool for measuring bone mass.

bones, including endocrine disorders such as hyperthyroidism, hyperparathyroidism, and Cushing's syndrome, as well as inflammatory diseases such as arthritis and ankylosing spondylitis

THE EVOLUTION OF BONE HEALTH

Evidence of osteoporosis has been found in the fossil remains of Neanderthals and other branches of the human evolutionary tree, but generally prehistoric hominids appear to have had a rather low incidence of bone loss compared to what we see in our species (*Homo sapiens*). Actually, there is a body of evidence that suggests that as meat eating increased, so did the height and general health of these hominids. Mind you, the meat they scavenged and hunted was rich in health-promoting fats such as omega-3 EFAs and contained relatively low amounts of saturated fats, omega-6 EFAs, and other fats that can erode health when overconsumed. (By contrast, because they are raised on grains rather than grass, most modern, domesticated meat animals tend to have higher levels of omega-6 EFAs and lower levels of heart-healthy omega-3 EFAs.) These early hominids also were generally more physically active than us. In short, their diet and physical activity patterns were basically in greater harmony with what we evolved to thrive on.

With the advent of agriculture, our diet and lifestyle patterns began deviating greatly from the healthier ones that preceded them. For example, with the introduction of cereals and grains (and then excessive consumption of them) came compromised calcium absorption: cereals and grains contain compounds called phytates that limit mineral absorption. A less physically vigorous lifestyle and less exposure to sunlight (which helps us create bone-building vitamin D) further impacted bone health. The health-eroding consequences of this trend have been confirmed by studies done of archaeological human remains from *every corner of the globe,* studies that demonstrate an increased evidence of poor dental health, iron-deficiency anemia, infection, and bone loss from the advent of agriculture onward.

Some experts have pointed out that protein, such as would come from a meat-rich diet, would actually promote calcium loss and thus undermine bone integrity. However, protein's effect apparently can be offset by the inclusion of an ample supply of foods that help the body retain calcium, such as fruits and vegetables. Most prehistoric peoples, it would seem, took in a ratio of meat to vegetables and fruits that favored bone building and preservation.

In addition to having an increasing reliance on grains and cereals, post-agricultural peoples also adopted other dietary practices that promoted calcium loss or otherwise compromised bone building and preservation. Among these was a shift from a high potassium–low sodium dietary pattern to its reverse. Sodium increases calcium excretion in the urine and is being increasingly acknowledged among medical and nutrition experts as a major player in promoting bone loss.

The intake of calcium and magnesium also changed over time, favoring the former over the latter. Pre-agricultural peoples generally took in calcium and magnesium at a ratio of one part calcium to one part magnesium. Today, we take in ratios that are considerably different from this ancient pattern, as high as three or four parts calcium to one part magnesium. When animals are placed on high-calcium, normal-magnesium diets, magnesium levels in their body plummet. So, what's so bad about this? After all, isn't more calcium better when it comes to building and preserving bone? According to many experts, when the ratio of calcium to magnesium drifts too far from the 1:1 pattern of our ancestors, bone loss is actually encouraged. How? Magnesium is important to bone density and the prevention of bone fractures and is integral to the prevention of certain forms of heart disease and other chronic "diseases of civilization" as well. When the level of magnesium in cells drops, people become hypomagnesic, which sets the stage for bone loss. Not surprisingly, a comprehensive 1995 review of published research clearly showed that postmenopausal women given supplemental magnesium over a two-year period experienced a significant increase in their bone-mineral density. However, a similar analysis of many studies on calcium supplementation and bone-mineral density produced ambiguous results.

While still controversial, it makes sense that dietary and physical activity patterns consistent with our evolved nature will probably produce more health benefits, including bone preservation, than a diet at odds with this nature. Recent scientific studies appear to bear this out. For example, in a fourteen-year study involving more than 80,000 women, Harvard Medical School researchers found that women with the highest protein intakes were 26 percent less likely than those who ate the least protein to develop ischemic heart disease. In addition, protein-rich diets were of benefit to these women. And in a 2004 study carried out at Utah State University to assess the role of protein intake on hip fractures in the elderly, scientists found that "higher total protein intake was associated with a reduced risk of hip fracture in men and women 50–69 years, but not in men and women 70–89 years of age. The association between dietary protein intake and risk of hip fracture may be modified by age. Our study supports the hypothesis that adequate dietary protein is important for optimal bone health in the elderly 50–69 years of age."

PREVENTING AND REVERSING BONE LOSS

The National Osteoporosis Foundation states, "Osteoporosis is largely preventable for most people. Prevention of this disease is

MK-7 and Bone Loss Prevention

Taking as little as 5 micrograms (mcg) daily of MK-7 should have a significant benefit in preventing bone loss. In fact, growing evidence suggest that taking MK-7 as early as adolescence may have significant long-term preventative benefits in both bone and cardiovascular health. Additionally, growing research clearly suggests that MK-7 is one of the leading safe contenders for reversing bone loss.

very important because, while there are treatments for osteoporosis, there is currently no cure." The National Institutes of Health (NIH) and most of the major osteoporosis research and education centers agree that there are several basic measures people should employ to help prevent osteoporosis.

1. Get enough calcium and vitamin D every day.

The genesis of osteoporosis lies, in part, in inadequate calcium intake. For this reason, it is important to take in sufficient calcium every day. For women, this is about 1,000 milligrams (mg) per day from ages nineteen to fifty, and 1,200 mg per day from age fifty-one on up, according to the NIH. Foods rich in calcium include dairy products of all kinds and nondairy foods such as legumes, leafy green vegetables, tofu, nuts, sardines and salmon, and tortillas made with limestone.

However, calcium is only one side of the equation, the other being getting enough vitamin D. When vitamin D levels are inadequate, a deficiency state may arise that contributes to osteoporosis by reducing calcium absorption. Osteopororsis is, in fact, a prime example of the long-term effects of a vitamin D deficiency.

Vitamin D exists in nature in several forms, each with a different level of biological activity. Most are inactive in the human body, with the exception of calciferol. Ordinarily, we get vitamin D through its production in skin exposed to sunlight and also by dietary intake of calcium-containing foods. Once vitamin D is made or taken in, it must be converted in the liver and kidneys into its active form, 1,25-dihydroxyvitamin D, which actually functions as a hormone insofar as it sends a message to the intestines to increase the absorption of calcium and phosphorus.

The major biological role of vitamin D in our bodies is to help maintain normal blood levels of calcium and phosphorus. By virtue of its active role in helping promote calcium absorption, vitamin D helps us form and maintain strong bones. In addition, vitamin D works together with a number of other vitamins, minerals, and hormones to promote bone mineralization. Without adequate vitamin D, children develop a bone-weakening condition called rickets and adults can wind up with a similar condition called osteomalacia.

Sun exposure provides most of us with all the vitamin D we need. Of course, we must make allowances for the intensity of sunlight where we live, the season and time of day, cloud cover, industrial pollution (smog), and the use of sunscreens. These all influence our exposure to ultraviolet (UV) rays and thus our body's ability to synthesize vitamin D. A totally overcast sky, for example, reduces the energy of UV rays by 50 percent, and shade reduces it by 60 percent. Topical sunscreens with a sun protection factor (SPF) of 8 or more will block UV rays that help the body produce vitamin D, although the risk of cancer and accelerated skin weathering from overexposure to UV radiation must surely be considered. Generally speaking, exposure of the face, arms, and back to sunlight for ten to fifteen minutes at least twice weekly is sufficient to create enough vitamin D to maintain health and facilitate calcium absorption. People who must limit sun exposure because of a family or personal history of skin cancer or other medical conditions or limitations must strive to make sure they get enough vitamin D through dietary sources, vitamin D–rich supplements such as cod liver oil, or both.

2. Eat lots of vitamin K–rich foods.

Vitamin K–rich foods include kale, spinach, lettuce, watercress, leeks, cabbage, Brussels sprouts, broccoli, cauliflower, green beans, peas, apple, eggplant, cereals, and soybeans.

3. Postmenopausal women should consult a physician to find out whether hormone replacement therapy is indicated.

According to many experts, hormone replacement therapy (HRT) is most effective against osteoporosis if initiated during the first five years after menopause begins. For this reason, many doctors recommend HRT for their menopausal and postmenopausal patients. However, HRT works against osteoporosis only for as long as a woman takes the estrogen; she loses this protection once she has stopped taking it.

It is estimated that HRT results in a 50 to 80 percent decrease in vertebral fractures and a 25 percent decrease in nonvertebral fractures with five years of use. On average, the researchers found that for every ten thousand women who take estrogen plus progestin for a year, five fewer cases of hip fractures will occur than in a comparable number of women who do not take hormones.

However, in a subsequent study called HERS (Heart Estrogen/Progestin Replacement Study), scientists found no evidence of the reduction of fracture incidence with HRT in older women. Most alarmingly, data from the Female Health Initiative (FHI) indicates that HRT increases the incidence of breast and endometrial cancer as well as the incidence of stroke, coronary artery disease, and other health challenges related to blood clots.

Is there an alternative to HRT? Several alternatives appear quite promising, including raloxifene, a drug that exerts an estrogen-like effect by attaching to estrogen receptors in bone and cardiovascular tissues. Unlike estrogen itself, raloxifene interacts with estrogen receptors only in bone and cardiovascular tissue, and not in the lining of the uterus (endometrium) and breast. And in a major clinical trial involving 601 postmenopausal women, raloxifene brought about a modest increase in bone mass density of 2.4 percent in the lumbar spine and 2.0 percent for the whole body over a two-year period. These changes persisted during the third year of the study, and chemical markers of bone turnover were reduced to the normal premenopausal range in raloxifene-treated females. Raloxifene also decreased the serum total cholesterol level in treated women.

4. Discuss the use of alendronate (Fosamax) with your healthcare practitioner.

Alendronate belongs to a group of nonhormonal drugs called biphosphonates that work to slow or halt bone loss. Scientists have found that alendronate binds to a compound called hydroxyapatite in bone and thereby inhibits the activity of bone-resorbing osteoclasts. When daily oral doses of alendronate (5 mg, 20 mg, or 40 mg over a six-week period) were taken by postmenopausal women as part of controlled studies, researchers noted that the drug brought about biochemical changes that are associated with a reduction of bone resorption. They also noted that long-term treatment of osteoporotic patients with alendronate (10 mg per day for up to five years) reduced the amount of bone-resorption-associated compounds excreted in urine to levels typically seen in healthy premenopausal women. Treatment of osteoporotic men with alendronate (10 mg per day for two years and 70 mg per week for one year) also showed significant reductions in urinary excretion of key bone-resorption compounds.

5. Do regular weight-bearing exercise such as dancing, walking, or climbing stairs.

Weight stimulates osteoblasts to build or shore up bone. In other words, weight-bearing exercises stimulate the growth of bone cells and, with a regular exercise schedule, can help keep your bones strong.

6. Don't smoke.

Smoking reduces blood flow to bones throughout the body and thus the amount of oxygen they receive. Various studies have shown that the bones of smokers heal at a far slower rate than those of nonsmokers. So, bones are probably weakened over a lifetime of smoking, increasing a smoker's chances of developing osteoporosis.

THE NOVEL ROLE OF VITAMIN K_2

Scientists have discovered three proteins in bone that depend on vitamin K for their function. One of these is osteocalcin, which is synthesized by bone-forming cells called osteoblasts. The production of osteocalcin is regulated by the active form of vitamin D, with vitamin K playing a crucial role in helping osteocalcin grab on to minerals like calcium. While the exact function of osteocalcin is not yet fully known, it is thought to be involved in bone mineralization.

The matrix Gla protein (MGP), which is found in bone, cartilage, and soft tissues, may be important in terms of keeping soft tissues, cartilage, and blood vessels from calcifying (hardening). As described earlier, vitamin K helps ensure that this protein is properly carboxylated. When MGP is undercarboxylated, the body's soft tissues are at risk of calcification. Dr. Cees Vermeer of the Department of Biochemistry at the University of Maastricht in the Netherlands, one of the world's leading scientific investigators and authorities on vitamin K, and a group of Japanese scientists reported in a 2004 study that "serum MGP levels are inversely correlated with the severity of CAC." CAC stands for coronary artery calcification, which means that the lower the level of MGP, the greater the severity of calcification in coronary arteries; and conversely, the higher the level of MGP, the lower the degree of calcification in coronary arteries will be. MGP also apparently helps facilitate normal bone growth and development.

The third protein dependent on vitamin K is anticoagulant protein S, which is synthesized by osteoblasts. However, the role of this protein in bone metabolism is unclear.

The role of the K family of vitamins in bone health is suggested by a number of published studies. In a Tufts University pilot study involving nine healthy men and women, researchers found that increasing the intake of vitamin K to four times the government daily value (DV; once known as recommended dietary allowance, or RDA) resulted in a significant increase in the percentage of calcium-saturated osteocalcin in the test subjects.

The Nurses' Health Study followed 72,000 women over the course of a decade. Researchers were able to show that women whose vitamin K intake was exceedingly low (in the bottom one-fifth of all the women) had a 30 percent higher risk of hip fracture than women with a higher intake of vitamin K. These findings dovetail with those of researchers at Harvard Medical School, who found that substantially increasing the daily intake of vitamin K reduced the risk of hip fractures (in at least some women). This idea received additional support from a separate study in which more than eight hundred elderly men and women who were part of the famous Framingham Heart Study were looked at in terms of vitamin K intake and their risk of hip fracture. It was found that the men and women who took the greatest amount of vitamin K through their diet had only 35 percent the risk of hip fracture experienced by those whose vitamin K intake was the lowest.

Men and women who took the greatest amount of vitamin K through their diet had only 35 percent the risk of hip fracture experienced by those whose vitamin K intake was the lowest.

Beginning in 2002, another study divided 188 postmenopausal women between fifty and sixty years of age into three groups and treated them for three years. One group received a placebo; a second group took 500 mg of calcium, 150 mg of magnesium, 10 mg of zinc, and 320 IU of vitamin D_3 every day; and a third group received the same supplements as the second group with the addition of 1 mg of vitamin K_1 daily. The group that received minerals and vitamin D_3 without vitamin K showed only fleeting benefits. In the group that received vitamin K, bone loss in the neck of the femur (the bone that connects the leg to the hip) was reduced by 35 to 40 percent compared with the group supplemented with minerals and vitamins but not vitamin K. The scientists involved, including vitamin K authority Vermeer, stated that by extrapolating from these results, one would anticipate that lifelong supplementation could postpone fractures by up to a decade.

In a study carried out at the Keio University School of Medicine in Japan, researchers conducted a clinical trial in which they compared the effects of etidronate (also known as EHDP), which regulates bone metabolism, and vitamin K_2 (menatetrenone) on bone mineral density (BMD) and the incidence of vertebral fractures in postmenopausal women with osteoporosis. In the study, seventy-two osteoporotic women, ages fifty-seven to seventy-eight, who had all been postmenopausal for five years or longer, were randomly divided into three groups. For fourteen days out of every three months, one group took etidronate (200 mg per day); a second group took vitamin K_2 (45 mg per day); and a third group took calcium lactate (2 g per day). The BMD of these women was assessed in their forearms by use of dual-energy x-ray absorptiometry prior to treatment and then at regular intervals thereafter. Researchers noted that there were no significant differences in age, body mass index, years since menopause, and initial BMD among the three groups of women.

When the study ended, the scientists found that the group that had received calcium lactate had experienced only a significant decrease in BMD, while the group taking vitamin K_2 had a significant increase in BMD compared with that in the calcium-only group. The group that received etidronate had a significant increase in BMD compared with that of the other two groups. When they looked at the frequency of bone fractures that occurred, the scientists concluded that "despite the lower increase in BMD produced by menatetrenone (vitamin K_2), this agent, as well as etidronate, may have the potential to reduce osteoporotic vertebral fractures in postmenopausal women with osteoporosis."

Vitamin K_2 protects bone-building osteoblasts from undergoing programmed cell death (apoptosis), while at the same time encouraging mature bone-demolishing osteoclasts to undergo apoptosis.

Other studies have shown that vitamin K_2 protects bone-building osteoblasts from undergoing programmed cell death (apoptosis), while at the same time encouraging mature bone-demolishing osteoclasts to undergo apoptosis. Vitamin K_2 also inhibits the formation of new osteoclasts and retards the production and bone-eroding activity of a hormonelike inflammatory compound called prostaglandin E2 (PGE2). In addition, vitamin K_2 has been found to play a role in preserving the spongy bone found at the ends of long bones, such as the femur in the legs, which tend to weaken and experience tissue loss with age or the development of osteoporosis.

DIET

In the United States, our calcium intake is one of the highest in the entire world, and yet we also sport one of the highest rates of osteoporosis. Why? One reason is dietary: the mineral content of our bones is dependent not just upon calcium intake but more important on how much goes in and how much goes out, or our net calcium balance. Nutritionists, dietitians, and other experts generally emphasize calcium intake and downplay calcium excretion.

The foods we eat influence our bodies' calcium levels, not just as a result of the calcium they contain but also because everything we eat affects the body's acid/base balance. Foods generate compounds that are generally either acidic or alkaline ("base"). Low-carbohydrate diets, for example, tend to load the body with acid-generating foods. When the net load from a given meal or snack weighs in on the acid side, this acid must be counteracted (or buffered) by base compounds from the alkaline stores in the body. The calcium in bones is the largest alkaline storehouse in the human body; it is tapped to offset a net acid load and then passed out of the body in the urine. So, if calcium intake is low and a large amount of calcium is pulled from bone, or if calcium intake is high and the outflow from bones is higher still, a gradual loss of bone will result.

The foods that yield the greatest acid load are cereal grains, salt, hard cheeses, meats, and legumes, while the sole producers of alkaline compounds are fruits and vegetables. Given the fact that the average American consumes a disproportionate amount of cereal grains, salty processed foods, fatty meats, and cheeses compared to his or her consumption of fruits and vegetables, most Americans have a net acid load, and this tends to promote bone demineralization. The solution to this problem is to try to curtail our intake of or even eliminate cereal grains, hard cheeses, and such, and replace them with an abundance of green vegetables and fruits. This will help shift the acid/base balance back to one that favors keeping calcium in the body as opposed to losing it.

Another player in the calcium-bone saga is magnesium, a mineral that appears to prevent bone fractures and has been shown to increase bone density. Unfortunately, most people consume a ratio of calcium to magnesium that is about as discordant with what is good for bone health as is their intake of acid/base foods. Researchers have found that in pre-agricultural societies the calcium to magnesium ratio was about 1:1, whereas today in the United States and throughout the West the dietary ratio runs as high as 4:1. This is complicated by the fact that a high dietary intake of calcium actually can facilitate a magnesium deficiency, even when normal levels of magnesium are consumed. So the trick then is to balance the calcium to magnesium ratio—to get the intake at or about 1:1.

Our ancestors evolved consuming a pre-agricultural diet (sometimes called a Stone Age or Paleolithic diet) that consisted of about 65 percent complex carbohydrates (vegetables and fruits) and about 35 percent protein and fats (game meat and nuts rich with omega-3 fatty acids). Again, the ancestral calcium to magnesium ratio was about 1:1. Then, about ten thousand years ago, humankind began domesticating plants and animals (agriculture) and with this developed a more sedentary lifestyle. People began relying on domesticated beef and cow's milk for sustenance. Cow's milk and other dairy products such as butter and yogurt generally have calcium to magnesium ratios of about 12:1. These dairy foods helped raise our ancestors' overall dietary calcium to magnesium ratio from 1:1 to 3:1 or even 4:1. Not unexpectedly, skeletal remains of these peoples often show greater tooth decay and bone loss than was true of people who died prior to the advent of agriculture. And not surprisingly, scientists experimenting with rats found that animals will develop clinical signs of a magnesium deficiency after only three weeks on a high-calcium, normal-magnesium diet. Thus, the overall thrust of the available evidence points to a need for striking a balance between calcium and magnesium intake (through diet and supplements).

A final player worth considering in terms of dietary prevention of bone loss is sodium. Prehistoric, pre-agricultural peoples evolved consuming foods low in sodium and high in potassium, a pattern that favored survival and thus was conserved down through the millennia. When sodium intake is high, high blood pressure often results, as does an increase in calcium excretion in the urine and, with this, bone loss. Many experts now consider a high intake of sodium as one of the single greatest dietary risk factors for developing osteoporosis.

BEST DIETARY SOURCES OF CALCIUM AND MAGNESIUM

Dairy products such as yogurt and cheese are the most common sources of calcium in the American diet, but calcium can also be found in many "pre-agricultural" foods, as can magnesium.

Food	Calcium Content
Tofu, with calcium sulfate (1/2 cup, cooked)	435 mg
Atlantic sardines, with bones, canned (3 oz)	325 mg
Pink salmon, with bones, canned (3 oz)	180 mg
Beans (great northern, navy, white; 1/2 cup, cooked)	60–80 mg
Orange (1 medium)	60 mg
Dark leafy greens (collards, mustard greens, spinach; 1/2 cup, cooked)	50–135 mg
Nuts (24 almonds or 8 Brazil nuts)	50–70 mg

Source: U.S. Department of Agriculture

Food	Magnesium Content
Pumpkin seeds (1 oz)	152 mg
Tofu, raw, regular (1/2 cup)	127 mg
Broccoli, cooked (2 large stalks)	120 mg
Spinach, cooked (1/2 cup)	79 mg
Swiss chard, cooked (1/2 cup)	76 mg
Tomato paste, canned (1/2 cup)	67 mg
Dock (sorrel), cooked (1/2 cup)	60 mg
Nuts and seeds, all types (1 oz)	60 mg (avg.)
Succotash, cooked (1/2 cup)	51 mg
Beet greens, cooked (1/2 cup)	49 mg
Artichoke, cooked (1 medium)	47 mg
Okra, cooked (1/2 cup)	46 mg
Acorn squash, baked (1/2 cup cubed)	43 mg
Purslane, cooked (1/2 cup)	39 mg
Chestnuts (1 oz)	9 mg

Source: http://lesann.tripod.com/magnesium%20rich%20foods.htm

NUTRITIONAL SUPPLEMENTS

Here are but a few of the supplement measures that have been proven to prevent and, in some instances, help reverse bone loss.

Vitamin K_2 (Menaquinone-7)

Many experts are suggesting upward of 1–5 mg daily.

Vitamin C

Esterified C (ester C) appears to be the form that is best absorbed and utilized. Many physicians recommend at least 500–1,000 mg per day.

Other Cutting-Edge Compounds for Preventing Bone Loss

- **Genistein:** Genistein is an isoflavone found in soy foods. In the body, a compound called interleukin 1-beta (IL1-beta) can stimulate osteoblasts to increase bone resorption. In one laboratory study, genistein suppressed bone resorption in cell cultures of osteoclasts exposed to IL1-beta.
- **Curcumin:** Curcumin is an antioxidant found in the spice turmeric. A wealth of studies have shown that inflammatory cytokines play a major role in the manufacture of bone-destroying osteoclasts (osteoclastogenesis), which leads to bone resorption. The activation of a the receptor called NF-kappa-B ligand (RANKL) plays a critical role in spurring on the creation of bone-demolishing osteoclasts, as does the activity of tumor necrosis factor (TNF). In laboratory studies, curcumin inhibited both RANKL and TNF osteoclast production.
- **Lactoferrin:** Lactoferrin is an iron-binding glycoprotein (carbohydrate-protein combination) present in human and cow's milk. When mouse bone marrow cultures were exposed to lactoferrin, the creation of new bone-demolishing osteoclasts (osteoclastogenesis) was decreased in step with increasing doses. What was especially compelling was that osteoclastogenesis was completely arrested by 100 mcg/ml of lactoferrin. Lactoferrin had no effect on bone resorption by isolated mature osteoclasts.
- **Policosanol:** Policosanol is a cholesterol-lowering drug isolated from sugarcane wax that inhibits cholesterol synthesis in the liver through indirect reduction in the activity of a key cholesterol-manufacturing enzyme called hydroxymethylglutaryl coenzyme A (HMG-CoA) reductase. When used in female rats whose ovaries had been removed (thus mimicking the postmenopause state), policosanol prevented bone loss and decreased bone resorption.
- **Onion:** When researchers added 1 gram of onion to the daily food given rats, they saw significant inhibition of bone resorption.

Vitamin D_3 (Cholecalciferol)

If you get fifteen minutes or more of sunlight exposure each day, your body probably makes enough vitamin D. However, people over the age of fifty have a higher risk of developing vitamin D deficiency and should consider taking 1,000 IU daily, in divided doses, with or after meals.

Calcium and Magnesium

Strive for the pre-agricultural 1:1 intake, such as 1,500 mg of each daily.

Zinc and Copper

Zinc helps premote mineral absorption and thus helps ensure that calcium gets into the body and is available for use in building bones. Since zinc can cause a loss of copper, and vice versa, zinc is often taken with copper. Copper plays a critical role in keeping collagen, the protein from which bone and connective tissue is built, in optimal form. Note that at least six months of treatment with a zinc/copper combination is required before any bone-fortifying impact is manifest. Zinc should not be taken in amounts greater than 50 mg daily, as this can have side effects such as reduced immune function and a lowering of the "good" cholesterol HDL (high-density lipoprotein) levels. Copper intake should not exceed 5 mg daily; avoid copper if you have hemochromatosis or Wilson's disease.

Manganese

Women with osteoporosis have decreased plasma levels of manganese and an enhanced plasma response to oral manganese. In one telltale study, healthy postmenopausal women who took manganese (5 mg per day), copper (2.5 mg per day), and zinc (15 mg per day) in combination with calcium (1,000 mg per day) experienced less spinal bone loss over a period of two years than women who took a calcium supplement only.

Boron

Several studies have shown that boron improves the absorption and utilization of calcium and magnesium, especially when combined with calcium, magnesium, and riboflavin (vitamin B_2). It is considered essential for the utilization of vitamin D, which, in turn, enhances the absorption of calcium. Recent research demonstrates that boron may be essential in the conversion of vitamin D to its active form. A supplement dose of 1.5–3.0 mg per day appears to be safe and effective.

EXERCISE

Humankind evolved in an environment in which physical agility, stamina, and fitness paid rich dividends in terms of survival and leaving behind viable offspring (the name of the game in evolution). Accordingly, physical exertion would be expected to have a positive impact on our physical health and even mood, and it does. For example, intense activity such as aerobic exercise has been found to improve the cardiovascular system, muscle strength, and flexibility. It also tends to increase artery size and elasticity and prevent plaque buildup and the formation of blood clots. Regular exercise has been shown to boost HDL ("good") cholesterol levels and lower both total cholesterol levels and blood pressure. The lungs also benefit insofar as physical exertion and exercise enhance the ability to breathe deeply, easily, and efficiently. Exercise burns fat and often alleviates stress. And it builds and preserves bone as well.

The ideal exercise program for bone health is to engage in weight-bearing exercises when young, as this pulls and pushes on bones and encourages them to be healthy and thick. Older people also benefit from bone-building exercise, but not to the same degree as younger folks. Those over thirty-five years of age, as well as those who have been sedentary for a long time or who have (or suspect they might have) a medical condition, would be wise to consult a physician concerning the kinds of exercise that will not compromise their health.

Exercise need not be regimented or ritualized, although many people probably do better on a program that requires adherence to a routine. In light of the fact that bone health benefits have been documented from low-impact activities such as walking up and down stairs, many "vehicle-dependent" people would do well to park their machines and take to foot. In Japan, daily physical exertion is part of life. Most Japanese, for example, use trains to get to and from work or school, which requires negotiating stairs and train platforms. This consistent, moderate physical activity may be part of the reason the Japanese have a very long average life span (eight-two years for men, eight-four years for women).

However, it must be noted that the prevalence of osteoporosis in the Japanese population is about one in ten people, which parallels the rate seen here in the United States. So, why aren't the more physically active Japanese enjoying a lower rate of osteoporosis than the less active Americans? Part of the answer may lie in the fact that many Japanese have a smaller bone structure than is typical of Americans. Also, the Japanese diet, while rich in vegetables and fruits plus fish rich in healthful fats, also includes the use of sodium-rich soy sauce with meals and frequent consumption of grains such as rice that interfere with mineral absorption. The Japanese consume almost as much alcohol per capita as Americans (1.84 gallons per year) but probably suffer more of a negative health impact (including bone loss) from it because so many Japanese lack an enzyme needed to break down alcohol. And six in ten Japanese men smoke. Again, all these factors promote bone loss. If the Japanese were to maintain their robust level of daily physical activity and concomitantly reduce those dietary and lifestyle factors that increase bone loss or otherwise compromise bone integrity, straightforward logic suggests that the prevalence of osteoporosis would decline.

In the United States, a diet at odds with our evolved nature and lack of physical activity predispose many to bone loss. Here,

Recommended Exercises for Bone Health

- Walking
- Hiking
- Racquet sports
- Jogging
- Dancing
- Cross-country skiing
- Climbing stairs

Jumping and running sports are also great exercises for bone health: basketball, volleyball, soccer, field hockey, and softball are good ways to build strong bones.

Source: National Institutes of Health (NIH), http://www.nichd.nih.gov/publications/pubs/boneup_boneloss.pdf

cars are virtually considered a necessity, physically taxing activity is minimized, and a great many people wind up as proverbial couch potatoes. So, why isn't the prevalence of osteoporosis higher? Part of the reason may lie in the general population being bigger boned and also heavier—weight on bones tends to build them up. But excess weight sets the stage for heart disease and certain cancers, so it is a poor substitute for a healthy, bone-health-promoting diet and lifestyle pattern.

Turning the tables on an inactive lifestyle need not involve grueling, boringly repetitive exercise but rather may be as simple as doing by choice what the Japanese do by design—climbing stairs and otherwise doing things that put some pressure and pull on your bones.

HORMONE REPLACEMENT THERAPY

When menopause begins, the ovaries cease to produce certain hormones, chief among them estrogen and progesterone, that drive the reproductive cycle. The loss of these hormones can cause a host of changes in women's bodies, resulting in conditions ranging from hot flashes and night sweats to, potentially, osteoporosis.

Hormone replacement therapy (HRT) is the administration of estrogen, often in combination with progesterone, to replace these reproductive hormones. HRT is approved by the U.S. Food and Drug Administration (FDA) for the prevention and treatment of osteoporosis in postmenopausal women.

HRT also helps women combat menopause-related thickening of the vagina, vaginal dryness, pain with intercourse, and loss of bladder control. Many doctors now prescribe forms of estrogen that affect only target tissues and that are not sent coursing throughout the user's body. HRT has also shown efficacy in decreasing the risk of hip fractures later in life. The loss of estrogen over time can lead to increased bone resorption as well as calcium loss from the kidneys, which increases the potential for bone loss and decreased bone density.

That said, it should be kept in mind that most studies of HRT were financed by private drug firms and involved the use of progestins and estrogens derived from the urine of mares (horses). Forms of these hormones that are identical to the natural forms found in humans have not been tested as extensively as the animal-derived forms. This disparity in the nature of the clinical trials is important, because the fact that so many studies found a downside to the use of animal estrogens and progestins does not necessarily mean that there is a downside to the use of the forms identical to those found in humans. At least one pilot study has confirmed this: a form of commonly used horse-derived estrogen called conjugated equine estrogen was found to be associated with an increased risk of clots in veins, while a form of nonanimal estrogen carried no such risk.

There is also evidence that oral forms of progestin and horse-derived estrogen pills can aggravate existing liver or gallbladder problems, cause blood clots, and may with prolonged use increase the risk of breast cancer. Use of horse-derived estrogen and progesterone appears to increase the risk of uterine cancers. This duo has also been shown to increase blood triglyceride levels, which can lead to various circulatory problems.

In 2002, the results of a major study by the Women's Health Initiative indicated that a combination of synthetic progestins and horse-urine-derived estrogen carried measured risks that outweighed measured benefits. In the double-blind study, which took place over five-plus years, 16,608 women, fifty to seventy-nine years old (sixty-three was the average age when the study began), were divided into two groups. One received a combination of progestins and estrogens (8,506 women) and the other a placebo (8,102 women). For women fifty to fifty-nine years old, there was a trend toward a reduced risk of cardiovascular disease in the hormone-supplemented group. However, the findings from other studies suggest that when horse-derived estrogens are taken orally, liver function is compromised in certain respects and with this the risk of blood clots increases. What is needed then is a comparison trial using the horse-derived hormones alongside forms of estrogen and progesterone that are identical to those found in humans, such as estradiol and estriol used as transdermal creams (applied to and absorbed through the skin).

Until a consensus is reached in the medical community, women would be well advised to discuss their individual circumstances with an informed physician who can help weigh risks versus benefits to determine whether HRT is a prudent course of action.

DRUGS AND OTHER COMPOUNDS

Calcitonin is a hormone manufactured in the thyroid gland that retards the breakdown of bone. Supplemental calcitonin is usually given as an injection or a nasal spray and is approved by the FDA for the treatment of osteoporosis in men and women. Calcitonin can also be obtained from natural sources such as salmon or made in the laboratory (synthetic). Although calcitonin is by and large considered safe, supplementation with it may not be as effective as other treatments for osteoporosis.

Raloxifene (Evista) is an oral drug that is approved by the FDA for the prevention and treatment of osteoporosis in postmenopausal women who are not undergoing hormone replacement therapy. Raloxifene belongs to a class of drugs called selective estrogen receptor modulators (SERMs), meaning that this compound attaches to cell receptors where estrogen usually binds. SERMs exert their estrogen-like effects in the bones and some other parts of the body, but not throughout the body like estrogen does.

Teriparatide (Forteo) is a relatively new drug approved by the FDA in 2002 for the treatment of osteoporosis. Teriparatide is a human parathyroid hormone (PTH) that is manufactured in bacteria that have been genetically altered (through recombinant DNA technology). In the body, PTH is naturally produced by the parathyroid gland, which straddles the thyroid, and it plays a crucial role in regulating the body's calcium levels. Teriparatide acts like natural PTH in that it increases bone formation by boosting the activity of bone-building osteoblasts. As a result, osteoblasts build up bone faster than osteoclasts can break it down, which favors boosts in bone density. Teriparatide is available only in injection form and can be used daily by postmenopausal women and also men at risk of experiencing osteoporotic fractures. At the time of publication, however, it cost $600 per month, thus making it very expensive compared with other drugs used to treat osteoporosis.

CONCLUSION

When it comes to maintaining your bone health, it's clear there are many important steps you can take, and supplementing with vitamin K_2, or specifically MK-7, is just one of them. Having read this chapter, you are much more familiar with what you can do to prevent bone loss. Taking supplemental K_2 is a great start, but don't stop there. Be sure to consider the other advice in this chapter as well.

Conclusion

People today generally live long lives, but many are struggling with chronic illnesses and health challenges, such as cardiovascular disease and other "diseases of civilization." Many of these are linked to the wear and tear associated with a long life, but unhealthy dietary choices, a lack of exercise, stress, and a multitude of other players give rise to or contribute to others.

A growing body of scientific evidence indicates that people in societies in which diet and exercise patterns mirror those of our Stone Age ancestors have few, if any, of these maladies. This strongly suggests that we can circumvent or ameliorate many of them by simply bringing our lifestyles into harmony with our evolved nature. The addition of foods and supplements rich in various antioxidants, B vitamins, s-adenosylmethionine (SAMe), and vitamin K_2, plus culinary spices such as cayenne, turmeric, and garlic and green, white, and black tea, can also help in this regard.

As this book has shown, the form of vitamin K_2 known as menaquinone-7 (MK-7) has proven effective in halting and reversing bone loss in both lab animals and humans. It has also proven effective in helping shuttle calcium out of hardened arteries for incorporation into bones or for excretion. Japan, in fact, has approved vitamin K_2 as a treatment of osteoporosis. And in the European Union, world-renowned vitamin K_2 researcher Dr. Cees Vermeer has shown through his clinical studies that MK-7 is a very effective intervention for addressing various heart and bone ailments. Vermeer's findings have been born out by studies published by scientists in many other countries.

Most of the MK-7 Americans get comes through their diet—a diet notoriously lacking foods rich in vitamin K_2, such as green leafy vegetables and soybean-based foods such as natto. Dietary change is needed, yes, but it may not be sufficient to ensure that the average person gets enough MK-7 to prevent bone loss and arterial calcification. Thankfully, MK-7 is now appearing in various other guises, including multivitamin formulas. Make sure that you and your family are getting enough of this vital form of vitamin K_2.

Glossary

Alendronate. A medication that belongs to a class of drugs known as bisphosphonates. It is approved by the FDA for the prevention and treatment of bone loss.

Atheroma. A buildup of fatty, fibrous, and other material on the walls of the arteries.

Atherosclerosis. The clogging, narrowing, and hardening of large arteries and medium-size blood vessels.

Bone resorption. The process whereby bone is dissolved and its constituent elements freed up and absorbed within the body.

Calcitonin. A hormone manufactured in and secreted by the thyroid that lowers calcium levels in the blood.

Carboxylation. The introduction of a carboxyl group (denoted in chemistry as -COOH) into a compound or molecule.

Coronary artery disease. The narrowing of the coronary arteries sufficient to prevent adequate blood supply to the heart muscle.

Cytokine. A small protein released by cells that exerts specific effects on the interactions between cells, on communication between cells, or on the activity of cells. The family of cytokines includes the interleukins, lymphokines, and cell-signaling molecules, such as tumor necrosis factor (TNF) and the interferons (interferons set off inflammation and help the body respond to infection).

Estrogen. A hormone produced by the ovaries and testes that plays a key role in the development of secondary sexual characteristics in men and women, induces menstruation in women, and protects against bone loss and certain brain and circulatory disorders (especially in women).

Fibrinogen. A protein involved in blood clotting (coagulation).

Fibrinolytic. Describes a compound that tends to act on fibrinogen in such a way as to prevent the formation of clots and to break up existing ones.

Forteo. *See* Teriparatide

Fosamax. *See* Alendronate

High-density lipoprotein (HDL). A protein in blood plasma that promotes the breakdown and removal of cholesterol from the body.

Hormone replacement therapy (HRT). The replacement of the female hormones estrogen and progestin (synthetic progesterone) in women who no longer produce these hormones due to removal of the ovaries or natural decline (menopause).

Isoflavone. An estrogen-like substance (phytoestrogen) made by some plants that weakly mimics the effects of estrogen in the human body.

Low-density lipoproteins (LDL). A complex of lipids and proteins that transports cholesterol in the body and tends to promote atherosclerosis (especially when oxidized).

Menaquinone 7 (MK-7). One of thirteen menaquinone compounds that make up vitamin K_2.

Monoamine oxidase inhibitors (MAOIs). A class of drugs employed by doctors to treat depression and migraine.

Monounsaturated fatty acid. An unsaturated fatty acid containing only one carbon-to-carbon double bond. Monounsaturated fats may result in reduced blood cholesterol levels, which, in turn, reduces the risk of developing heart disease.

Omega-3 fatty acid. Any of several polyunsaturated fatty acids, found in leafy green vegetables, vegetable oils, and fish such as salmon, that have proven effective in reducing serum cholesterol levels and preventing the formation of blood clots.

Omega-6 fatty acids. A type of polyunsaturated fatty acid found in abundance in protein and most seed oils. These fats are health-promoting as long as their intake is well below that of omega-3 fatty acids.

Osteoblasts. Cells whose function is to form the tissue and minerals that give bone its strength.

Osteocalcin. The major (non-collagen-based) protein of the bone matrix; it is synthesized by osteoblasts.

Osteoclasts. Cells that break down bone.

Osteoporosis. A decrease in bone mass and density that carries with it an increased risk and/or incidence of fracture.

Oxidation. The process of combining oxygen with another substance leading to chemical changes in which atoms lose electrons.

Parathyroid hormone. A hormone made by the parathyroid gland that helps the body store and use calcium.

Polyphenols. A class of chemicals made and stored in plants (phytochemicals) that mop up cell-damaging free radicals and are found in high concentrations in green tea. They are associated with the prevention of cancer and heart disease.

Polyunsaturated fatty acid. A fatty acid derived from plant and some animal sources such as fish that is liquid at room temperature and contains more than one carbon-to-carbon double bond. Unsaturated fats help reduce blood cholesterol levels.

Progesterone. A female steroid hormone produced and secreted by the ovaries and also synthesized in large amounts by the placenta during pregnancy.

Raloxifene. A selective estrogen receptor modulator (SERM) drug that slows bone loss.

Saturated fat. Fats that are usually solid or almost solid at room temperature. All animal fats and dairy products contain saturated fats, as do some vegetable oils such as palm, palm kernel, and coconut oils. Fats containing mostly unsaturated fat can be made more saturated through a process called hydrogenation, which is used to create many margarines. Saturated fats cause the body to produce more cholesterol, which, in turn, may raise blood cholesterol levels.

Soy isoflavone. *See* Isoflavone

Triglycerides. The body's storage form for fat; as such, most triglycerides are found in adipose (fat) tissue. Some triglycerides circulate in the blood to provide fuel for muscles, but in excess they can contribute to vascular disease.

Teriparatide. Lab-manufactured human parathyroid hormone.

Viscosity. The thickness or resistance to flow of a liquid.

Vitamin D_3 (cholecalciferol). A vitamin produced by the body when exposed to ultraviolet light; also obtained from dietary sources. Vitamin D_3 is a hormone that has an important role in calcium and phosphorus metabolism.

Vitamin K. One of two naturally occurring fat-soluble vitamins (vitamin K_1 and K_2) that are needed to maintain normal blood clotting and have also been shown to help prevent osteoporosis and calcification of blood vessels. Vitamin K_1 is made by plants; vitamin K_2 is found in certain foods and is made by bacteria in the human gut and in fermentation tanks in laboratories.

Resources

Vitamin K2 and MK-7 Supplements

The market for vitamin K2 and MK-7 is rapidly growing. Keep a watchful eye out for supplement companies that offer MK-7 and vitamin K2, either individually or as part of a targeted formula. Your local retailer can tell you which formulas contain these important compounds. The following is a sampling of the currently available sources for vitamin K2 and MK-7 products.

Jarrow Formulas, Inc.
1824 South Robertson Blvd
Los Angeles, CA 90035
www.jarrow.com
Offers Jarrow brand products.

Whole Foods Market
Stores available throughout the United States.
www.wholefoodsmarket.com
Offers a variety of nutritional products.

Wild Oats Natural Market Place
Stores available throughout the United States
www.wholefoodsmarket.com
Offers a variety of nutritional products.

Additional Information on Vitamin K

Linus Pauling Institute
Oregon State University
Website: http://lpi.oregonstate.edu/
Vitamin K link: http://lpi.oregonstate.edu/infocenter/vitamins/vitaminK/index.html

Heart Disease Risk and Rates

To take a free online interactive test to assess your risk of developing heart disease, go to Harvard Univeristy's "Your Disease Risk" website at http://www.yourdiseaserisk.harvard.edu/, and click on the "Heart Disease" button.

For additional information on heart disease, visit the American Heart Association at www.americanheart.org.

Osteoporosis Risk and Rates

To take a free online interactive test to assess your risk of developing osteoporosis, go to Harvard University's "Your Disease Risk" website at http://www.yourdiseaserisk.harvard.edu and click on the "Osteoporosis" button.

Osteoporosis rates worldwide, by region and constituent countries, are available online at http://www.osteofound.org/press_centre/fact_sheet.html.

Paleolithic (Stone Age) Diet

Readers interested in learning more about the Paleolithic or Stone Age diet are urged to consult Dr. Loren Cordain's excellent book, *The Paleo Diet: Lose Weight and Get Healthy by Eating the Food You Were Designed to Eat* (Wiley, 2002).

Also recommended are the following:

- The PaleoDiet.com website, at http://paleodiet.com, which has a wealth of material, both popular and scientific
- "Introduction to the Paleolithic Diet," by Dr. Ben Balzer, available online at http://www.earth360.com/diet_paleodiet_balzer.html
- "Cave Men Diets Offer Insights to Today's Health Problems, Study Shows," from *Science Daily* (February 5, 2002), available online at http://www.sciencedaily.com/releases/2002/02/020205080142.htm.

References

Bharti, A. C., Y. Takada, and B. B. Aggarwal. "Curcumin (Diferuloylmethane) Inhibits Receptor Activator of NF-kappa B Ligand-induced NF-kappa B Activation in Osteoclast Precursors and Suppresses Osteoclastogenesis." *Journal of Immunology* 172, no. 10 (2004): 5940–5947.

Braam, L. A. J., M. H. J. Knapen, P. Geusens, et al. "Vitamin K_1 Supplementation Retards Bone Loss in Postmenopausal Women Between 50 and 60 Years of Age." *Calcification of Tissue International* 72 (2003; e-publication).

Cappuccio, F. P. "Dietary Prevention of Osteoporosis: Are We Ignoring the Evidence?" *American Journal of Clinical Nutrition* 63 (1996): 787–788.

Cauley, J. A., D. M. Black, E. Barrett-Connor, et al. "Effects of Hormone Replacement Therapy on Clinical Fractures and Height Loss: The Heart and Estrogen/Progestin Replacement Study (HERS)." *American Journal of Medicine* 110, no. 6 (2001): 442–450.

Cordain, Loren, Ph.D. "Are Higher Protein Intakes Responsible for Excessive Calcium Excretion?" Active Low-Carber Forums (1999). http://forum.lowcarber.org/archive/index.php/t-52311.

Cornish, J., K. E. Callon, D. Naot, et al. "Lactoferrin Is a Potent Regulator of Bone Cell Activity and Increases Bone Formation In Vivo." *Endocrinology* 145, no. 9 (2004): 4366–4374.

Delmas, P. D., N. H. Bjarnason, B. H. Mitlak, et al. "Effects of Raloxifene on Bone Mineral Density, Serum Cholesterol Concentrations, and Uterine Endometrium in Postmenopausal Women." *New England Journal of Medicine* 337, no. 23 (1997): 1641–1647.

Devine, A., R. A. Criddle, I. M. Dick, et al. "A Longitudinal Study of the Effect of Sodium and Calcium Intakes on Regional Bone Density in Postmenopausal Women." *American Journal of Clinical Nutrition* 62 (1995): 740–745.

Dhore, C. R., J. P. Cleutjens, E. Lutgens, et. al. "Differential Expression of Bone Matrix Regulatory Proteins in Human Atherosclerotic Plaques." *Arteriosclerosis Thrombosis and Vascular Biology* 21, no. 12 (2001): 1998–2003.

Evans, G. H., C. M. Weaver, D. D. Harrington, C. F. Babbs Jr. "Association of Magnesium Deficiency with the Blood-lowering Effects of Calcium." *Journal of Hypertension* 8 (1990): 327–337.

Favus, M. J., and S. Christakos. *Primer on the Metabolic Bone Diseases and Disorders of Mineral Metabolism.* 3rd ed. Philadelphia: Lippincott-Raven, 1996.

Feskanich, D., P. Weber, W. C. Willett, et al. "Vitamin K Intake and Hip Fractures in Women: A Prospective Study." *American Journal of Clinical Nutrition* 69, no. 1 (1999): 74–79.

Freeland-Graves, J., and C. Llanes. "Models to Study Manganese Deficiency." In *Manganese in Health and Disease,* edited by D. L. Klimis-Tavantzis. Boca Raton, FL: CRC Press, 1994.

Goldring, S. R., S. Krane, and L. V. Avioli. "Disorders of Calcification: Osteomalacia and Rickets." In *Endocrinology,* 3rd ed., 1204–1227. Philadelphia: W. B. Saunders, 1995.

Hara, K., Y. Akiyama, T. Nakamura, et al. "The Inhibitory Effect of Vitamin K_2 (Menatetrenone) on Bone Resorption May Be Related to Its Side Chain." *Bone* 16 (1995): 179–184.

Hara, K., Y. Akiyama, T. Tajima, M. Shiraki. "Menatetrenone Inhibits Bone Resorption Partly through Inhibition of PGE2 Synthesis In Vitro." *Journal of Bone and Mineral Research* 8 (1993): 535–542.

Heaney, R. P. "Long-latency Deficiency Disease: Insights from Calcium and Vitamin D." *American Journal of Clinical Nutrition* 78 (2003): 912–919.

Holick, M. F. "McCollum Award Lecture, 1994: Vitamin D: New Horizons for the 21st Century." *American Journal of Clinical Nutrition* 60 (1994): 619–630.

Holick, M. F. "Vitamin D: The Underappreciated D-lightful Hormone That Is Important for Skeletal and Cellular Health." *Current Opinion in Endocrinology and Diabetes* 9 (2002): 87–98.

Hu, Frank B., M. J. Stampfer, J. E. Manson, et al. "Dietary Protein and Risk of Ischemic Heart Disease in Women." *American Journal of Clinical Nutrition* 70, no. 2 (1999): 221–227.

Institute of Medicine, Food and Nutrition Board. *Dietary Reference Intakes: Calcium, Phosphorus, Magnesium, Vitamin D and Fluoride.* Washington, DC: National Academy Press, 1999.

Iwamoto, J., T. Takeda, and S. Ichimura. "Effect of Menatetrenone on Bone

Mineral Density and Incidence of Vertebral Fractures in Postmenopausal Women with Osteoporosis: A Comparison with the Effect of Etidronate." *Journal of Orthopedic Science* 6, no. 6 (2001): 487–492.

Iwasaki, Y., H. Yamato, H. Murayama, et al. "Menatetrenone Prevents Osteoblast Dysfunction in Unilateral Sciatic Neurectomized Rats." *Japanese Journal of Pharmacology* 90 (2002): 88–93.

Jodar Gimeno, E., M. Munoz-Torres, F. Escobar-Jimenez, et al. "Identification of Metabolic Bone Disease in Patients with Endogenous Hyperthyroidism: Role of Biological Markers of Bone Turnover." *Calcification of Tissue International* 61, no. 5 (1997): 370–376.

Jono, S., Y. Ikari, C. Vermeer, et al. "Matrix Gla Protein Is Associated with Coronary Artery Calcification as Assessed by Electron-beam Computed Tomography." *Thrombosis and Haemostasis* 91, no. 4 (2004): 790–794.

Kaneki, M., S. J. Hedges, T. Hosoi, et al. "Japanese Fermented Soybean Food as the Major Determinant of the Large Geographic Difference in Circulating Levels of Vitamin K_2: Possible Implications for Hip-fracture Risk." *Nutrition* 17, no. 4 (2001): 315–321.

Kaneki, M., Y. Mizuno, T. Hosoi, et al. "Serum Concentration of Vitamin K in Elderly Women with Involutional Osteoporosis." *Nippon Ronen Igakkai Zasshi* 32, no. 3 (1995): 195–200.

Kawata, T., J. H. Zernik, T. Fujita, et al. "Mechanism in Inhibitory Effects of Vitamin K_2 on Osteoclastic Bone Resorption: In Vivo Study in Osteoporotic (Op/op) Mice." *Journal of Nutrition Sci Vitaminol* 45 (1999): 501–507.

Koshihara, Y., K. Hoshi, M. Shiraki. "Vitamin K_2 (Menatetrenone) Inhibits Prostaglandin Synthesis in Cultured Human Osteoblast-like Periosteal Cells by Inhibiting Prostaglandin H Synthase Activity." *Biochemistry and Pharmacology* 46 (1993): 1355–1362.

Larsen, C. S. "Animal Source Foods and Human Health during Evolution." *Journal of Nutrition* 133, no. 11, suppl. 2 (2003): S3893–S3897.

Li, B. B., S. F. Yu, and S. Z. Pang. "Genistein Inhibits the Promotive Effect of IL-1beta on Osteoclastic Bone Resorption." *Beijing Da Xue Xue Bao* 36, no. 6 (2004): 642–645.

Lindeberg, S. "Apparent Absence of Cerebrocardiovascular Disease in Melanesians. Risk Factors and Nutritional Considerations—The Kitava Study." M.D., Ph.D. thesis, University of Lund, 1994. (A summary is available online as "On the Benefits of Ancient Diets" at www.paleodiet.com/lindeberg.)

Luft, F. C., U. Ganten, D. Meyer, et al. "Effect of High Calcium Diet on Magnesium, Catecholamine, and Blood Pressure of Stroke-prone Spontaneously Hypertensive Rats." *Proceedings of the Society for Experimental Biology and Medicine* 187 (1988): 474–481.

Macdonald, H. M., S. A. New, W. D. Fraser, et al. "Low Dietary Potassium Intakes and High Dietary Estimates of Net Endogenous Acid Production Are Associated with Low Bone Mineral Density in Premenopausal Women and Increased Markers of Bone Resorption in Postmenopausal Women." *American Journal of Clinical Nutrition* 81, no. 4 (2005): 923–933.

Manolagas, S. C., and R. L. Jilka. "Bone Marrow, Cytokines, and Bone Remodeling: Emerging Insights into the Pathophysiology of Osteoporosis." *New England Journal of Medicine* 332, no. 5 (1995): 305–311.

Mawatari, T., H. Miura, H. Higaki, et al. "Effect of Vitamin K_2 on Three-dimensional Trabecular Microarchitecture in Ovariectomized Rats." *Journal of Bone and Mineral Research* 15 (2000): 1810–1817.

Monetini, L., M. G. Cavallo, S. Manfrini, et al. "Antibodies to Bovine Beta-casein in Diabetes and Other Autoimmune Diseases." *Hormone and Metabolism Research* 34, no. 8 (2002): 455–459.

Nestel, P., H. Shige, S. Pomeroy, et al. "The n-3 Fatty Acids Eicosapentaenoic Acid and Docosahexaenoic Acid Increase Systemic Arterial Compliance in Humans." *American Journal of Clinical Nutrition* 76 (2002): 326–330.

Noa, M., R. Mas, S. Mendoza, et al. "Policosanol Prevents Bone Loss in Ovariectomized Rats." *Drugs Experimental and Clinical Research* 30, no. 3 (2004): 117–123.

Nordin, B. E. C., A. G. Need, H. A. Morris, M. Horowitz. "The Nature and Significance of the Relationship between Urinary Sodium and Urinary Calcium in Women." *Journal of Nutrition* 123 (1993): 1615–1622.

Parfitt, A. M. "Osteomalacia and Related Disorders." In *Metabolic Bone Disease and Clinically Related Disorders,* 2nd ed., edited by L. V. Avioli and S. M. Krane, 329–396. Philadelphia: W. B. Saunders, 1990.

Scarabin, P. Y., E. Oger, and G. Plu-Bureau. "Estrogen and Thrombo-Embolism Risk Study Group, Differential Association of Oral and Transdermal Oestrogen-replacement Therapy with Venous Thrombo- embolism Risk." *Lancet* 362, no. 9382 (2003): 428–432.

Schurgers, L. J., P. E. Dissel, H. M. Spronk, et al. "Role of Vitamin K and Vitamin K–dependent Proteins in Vascular Calcification." *Zeitschrift fur Kardiologie* 90, suppl. 3 (2001): 57–63.

Seelig, M. S., Heggtveit H. A. "Magnesium Interrelationships in Ischemic Heart Disease: A Review." *American Journal of Clinical Nutrition* 27 (1974): 59–79.

Shearer, M. J. "Role of Vitamin K and Gla Proteins in the Pathophysiology of Osteoporosis and Vascular Calcification." *Current Opinion in Clinical Nutrition and Metabolism Care* 3, no. 6 (2000): 433–438.

Silagy, C., and A. Neil. "Garlic as a Lipid Lowering Agent: A Meta-analysis." *Journal of the Royal College of Physicians London* 28, no. 1 (1994): 39–45.

Sojka, J. E., and C. M. Weaver. "Magnesium Supplementation and Osteoporosis." *Nutrition Reviews* 53 (1995): 71–74.

Strause, L., P. Saltman, K. T. Smith, et al. "Spinal Bone Loss in Postmenopausal Women Supplemented with Calcium and Trace Minerals." *Journal of Nutrition* 124, no. 7 (1994): 1060–1064.

Tamatani, M., S. Morimoto, M. Nakajima, et al. "Decreased Circulating Levels of Vitamin K and 25-Hydroxyvitamin D in Osteopenic Elderly Men." *Metabolism* 47, no. 2 (1998): 195–199.

Tintut, Y., and L. L. Demer. "Recent Advances in Multifactorial Regulation of Vascular Calcification." *Current Opinion in Lipidology* 12, no. 5 (2001): 555–560.

Tsukamoto, Y. "Studies on Action of Menaquinone-7 in Regulation of Bone Metabolism and Its Preventive Role of Osteoporosis." *Biofactors* 22, no. 1–4 (2004): 5–19.

van den Berg, H. "Bioavailability of Vitamin D." *European Journal of Clinical Nutrition* 51:Suppl 1 (1997): S76–S79.

Varo, P. "Mineral Element Balance and Coronary Heart Disease." *International Journal for Vitamin and Nutrition Research* 44 (1974): 267–273.

Visudhiphan. S., S. Poolsuppasit, O. Pibolnukarintr, et al. "The Relationship between High Fibrinolytic Activity and Daily Capsicum Ingestion in Thais." *American Journal of Clinical Nutrition* 35 (1982): 1452–1458.

Wengreen, H. J., R. G. Munger, N. A. West, et al. "Dietary Protein Intake and Risk of Osteoporotic Hip Fracture in Elderly Residents of Utah." *Journal of Bone and Mineral Research* 19, no. 4 (2004): 537–545.

Wetli, H. A., R. Brenneisen, I. Tschudi, et al. "A Gamma-glutamyl Peptide Isolated from Onion (*Allium cepa L.*) by Bioassay-guided Fractionation Inhibits Resorption Activity of Osteoclasts." *Journal of Agriculture Food and Chemistry* 53, no. 9 (2005): 3408–3414.

Yamaguchi, M., and Z. J. Ma. "Inhibitory Effect of Menaquinone-7 (Vitamin K_2) on Osteoclast-like Cell Formation and Osteoclastic Bone Resorption in Rat Bone Tissues In Vitro." *Molecular and Cellular Biochemistry* 228, no. 1–2 (2001): 39–47.

Yamaguchi, M., E. Sugimoto, and S. Hachiya. "Stimulatory Effect of

Menaquinone-7 (Vitamin K_2) on Osteoblastic Bone Formation In Vitro." *Molecular and Cellular Biochemistry* 223, no. 1–2 (2001): 131–137.

Yamaguchi, M., H. Taguchi, Y. H. Gao, et al. "Effect of Vitamin K_2 (Menaquinone-7) in Fermented Soybean (Natto) on Bone Loss in Ovariectomized Rats." *Journal of Bone and Mineral Metabolism* 17, no. 1 (1999): 23–29.

Yamaguchi, M., S. Uchiyama, and Y. Tsukamoto. "Inhibitory Effect of Menaquinone-7 (Vitamin K_2) on the Bone-resorbing Factors-induced Bone Resorption in Elderly Female Rat Femoral Tissues In Vitro." *Molecular Chemistry and Biochemistry* 245, no. 1–2 (2003): 115–120.

Yamaguchi, M., S. Uchiyama, and Y. Tsukamoto. "Stimulatory Effect of Menaquinone-7 on Bone Formation in Elderly Female Rat Femoral Tissues In Vitro: Prevention of Bone Deterioration with Aging." *International Journal of Molecular Medicine* 10, no. 6 (2002): 729–733.

Index

About the Authors

Larry Howard has an A.E. degree in teacher's education from Fullerton College and a B.S. in physical education with an emphasis in special education from California State University–Fullerton, and he completed his internship in special education through California State University–Los Angeles. For several years, he worked as a teacher and adjunctive therapist. He left academia to become a seminar speaker, marketing consultant, vice president, and ultimately president of companies specializing in nutritional and fortified food products. Since 2000, he has created, patented, and implemented nutritional therapies for pain, drug addiction, and depression. He is also one of the leaders in sourcing and importing well-researched drugs that are available by prescription in Europe but are considered natural compounds in the United States.

Anthony G. Payne is staff biological theoretician and a senior science writer at the Steenblock Research Institute a 501c3 nonprofit organization located in San Clemente, California. He holds undergraduate and graduate degrees in biological anthropology (B.S., M.A.), plus a doctorate in nutritional medicine from Aksem Oriental Medical School in Manila, Philippines. Dr. Payne has been doing bench research and product development for numerous firms, such as BioProducts Inc., PCT Company Inc., Pacific Biologic, and Inter-Cal Inc., since 1985. From the late 1980s through the 1990s, he served on staff at an integrative medical clinic, on the board of scientific advisers to the Earthrise Corporation, and as interim superintendent of education for the Orthodox Catholic Education System. Dr. Payne then taught at two universities and numerous private institutes in Japan (1999–2003). In 1996 he was awarded an honorary M.D. and two international gold medals in science and medicine by Open International University for his work on eradicating solid tumors by manipulating critical metabolic pathways. Dr. Payne is a member of the Choctaw Nation of Oklahoma (www.choctawnation.com) and a twenty-plus-year member of Mensa. He is also the author of numerous articles and papers and is coauthor (with Dr. David Steenblock) of *Umbilical Cord Stem Cell Therapy: The Gift of Healing from Healthy Newborns* (Basic Health Publications, 2006). A sampling of Dr. Payne's writings can be found online at http://14ushop.com/wizard. He and his wife, Sachi, live in Southern California. He can be reached by e-mail at biotheoretician@gmail.com.